HOMEOPATHY
FOR
HEADACHES

BOOK YOUR PLACE ON OUR WEBSITE AND MAKE THE READING CONNECTION!

We've created a customized website just for our very special readers, where you can get the inside scoop on everything that's going on with Zebra, Pinnacle and Kensington books.

When you come online, you'll have the exciting opportunity to:

- View covers of upcoming books
- Read sample chapters
- Learn about our future publishing schedule (listed by publication month *and author*)
- Find out when your favorite authors will be visiting a city near you
- Search for and order backlist books from our online catalog
- Check out author bios and background information
- Send e-mail to your favorite authors
- Meet the Kensington staff online
- Join us in weekly chats with authors, readers and other guests
- Get writing guidelines
- AND MUCH MORE!

Visit our website at http://www.kensingtonbooks.com

HOMEOPATHY
FOR
HEADACHES

Ursula Stone

Kensington Books
Kensington Publishing Corp.
http://www.kensingtonbooks.com

KENSINGTON BOOKS are published by

Kensington Publishing Corp.
850 Third Avenue
New York, NY 10022

Kensington and the K logo Reg. U.S. Pat. & TM Off.

First Printing: May, 1999
10 9 8 7 6 5 4 3 2

Printed in the United States of America

DISCLAIMER

This book is intended as a source of information for headache sufferers. Every effort has been made to include the most up-to-date and accurate information; however, it is impossible to include everything in a basic guide, and there can be no guarantee that this information won't change in time as a result of ongoing medical research.

All matters regarding your health require medical supervision. The information presented herein is intended to supplement, not replace, the medical advice of trained professionals. Before you adopt any of the ideas, procedures, or suggestions contained in this book, consult your own physician to make sure that they are appropriate for you.

Any adoption of the information herein is at the reader's discretion. Neither the author nor the publisher assume any responsibility or liability arising directly or indirectly from the use of the information in this book.

The highest ideal of cure is rapid, gentle and permanent restoration of the health, or removal and annihilation of the disease in its whole extent, in the shortest, most reliable, and most harmless way, on easily comprehensible principles.

—Dr. Samuel Hahnemann

Homeopathy is one of the rare medical approaches which carries no penalties—only benefits.

—Yehudi Menuhin, violinist and
Past President of the
Hahnemann Society, U.K.

Homeopathy cures a greater number of cases than any other method of treatment.

—Mahatma Gandhi

You may honestly feel grateful that homeopathy has survived the attempts of the allopathists (orthodox physicians) to destroy it.

—Mark Twain

To like things like, whatever one may ail; there is certain help.

—Johann Wolfgang von Goethe, *Faust*

Through the like, disease is produced, and through the application of the like it is cured.

—Hippocrates

Contents

Part Two: Headache

PART THREE: THE MATERIA MEDICA, A CATALOG OF REMEDIES

PART FOUR: ADDITIONAL INFORMATION

INTRODUCTION

Homeopathy was introduced in the United States in the 1820s by a German doctor, Constantine Hering. In 1844, the first national medical association in the United States, the American Institute of Homeopathy, was founded. By the turn of the twentieth century, almost one quarter of all doctors were practicing homeopathy, and there were 22 homeopathic schools throughout the country in cities such as Chicago, Philadelphia, and Ann Arbor.

The discovery and widespread use of antibiotics eclipsed homeopathy, and, by the 1920s, its practice was largely abandoned in America. (It continued to flourish in Europe, however, especially in England.) The remedies were given legal status in 1938 and their manufacture and distribution is still governed by the FDA. So, although there are no accredited training programs solely in homeopathy in the United States, anyone who is trained and licensed as a health care practitioner and has authority to prescribe medicines can prescribe homeopathic remedies as part of his medical practice. Certification programs, some of which are quite rigorous, are not accredited. People who learn homeopathy through these programs, but are not licensed health care practitioners, can be helpful as consultants. They can assist you or your doctor in identifying useful remedies. Homeopathy can be a beneficial adjunct to conventional medicine—remedies can be used to alleviate the side effects of chemotherapy or radiation treatment, to help the body clear anesthesia after surgery, or to help bones heal after a fracture.

If you decide to try homeopathy, you should limit it to self-care for non-life-threatening, acute illnesses—colds, headaches, or upset stomachs, for example—and injuries such as sprains, bruises, and cuts that don't require stitches. Severe or chronic illnesses and injuries should always be evaluated and monitored by a doctor.

Homeopathy is an art as much as it is a science. It is important to work with someone who is experienced as well as trained in the practice, someone whom you trust, and with whom you can be absolutely frank about the totality of your health. The Resources section in the back of this book lists a variety of organizations that can provide you with more information or help you locate a reputable practitioner.

PART ONE

HOMEOPATHY

FREQUENTLY ASKED QUESTIONS

What is homeopathy?

Homeopathy is a medical system that treats illness and injury with specially prepared substances called remedies. The root words *homeo* and *pathy* mean "similar suffering" and reflect the foremost idea in the treatment philosophy, usually stated as "like cures like." The guiding principles of homeopathy—like cures like, minimal doses, single medicines, and prescribing based on an assessment of the totality of symptoms—were established by its founder Dr. Samuel Hahnemann and form an effective, cohesive philosophy that has remained unchanged for more than 100 years.

The remedies, most of which are derived from plants, can be used to treat or to augment treatment for the full range of human ailments from a simple cold or sprained ankle to terminal illnesses and mental health.

As with any medical system, however, some conditions can be treated safely at home, while others are best left to the care of trained and experienced professionals. Persistent, severe, or recurring conditions should be eval-

uated and treated by your physician and, if you choose
to augment that treatment, by an experienced homeopath.
Before undertaking any medical therapy, discuss it with
your doctor and your homeopath. And once the treatment
is under way, keep both of them informed about any
reactions that result.

How did it get started?

Samuel Hahnemann (1755–1843), a German doctor and
chemist, founded homeopathy. He defined its philosophy
and procedures in a book called *Organon of Medicine*.
("Organon" is a term used in philosophy for a set of
logical requirements for scientific demonstration, or a
body of principles of scientific or philosophic investigation.) Hahnemann began the research and experiments
that homeopathy is based on in 1790; he continued to
refine the principles and practice of homeopathy throughout his long life. He revised his *Organon of Medicine* for
the sixth and last time before his death at age 83.

Dr. Hahnemann enjoyed an early and successful career
practicing the standard medicine of his day, even serving
as personal physician to some of Germany's royal court.
Nevertheless, he saw that the medicine he practiced—
bloodletting and cathartic dosing with mercury, arsenic,
sulfur, belladonna, and other toxic chemicals—often did
more harm than good. Disenchanted with medicine, he
retired from practice. To support his family, he turned a
gift for languages into a successful career as a translator
of medical and scientific material.

While translating a work by a noted physiologist, he
was startled by the doctor's assertion that Peruvian bark
(cinchona, a source of quinine) was effective against
malaria because it was bitter and astringent. Ever the
scientist, Hahnemann made a concoction that was even

more bitter and astringent than Peruvian bark, then demonstrated that it was useless against malaria. The curative property, he now knew, lay elsewhere. Intrigued, he began taking small quantities of Peruvian bark and soon began to suffer with a persistent headache and cyclic chills, fever, and sweats—the classic symptoms of malaria. This physiological reaction sparked an intuitive leap: Hahnemann wondered if there might be a connection between the bark's ability to provoke a healthy body into counterfeiting malaria and its efficacy in curing it.

He gathered a group of people willing to help him test his idea and began a series of provings (what are now called clinical trials) in which he and they ingested small quantities of various "medicines" and kept meticulous records about their physical condition. When Dr. Hahnemann gathered these records together and analyzed them, he found that when healthy people take particular medicines, they generate symptoms that mirror the illness for which the medicine is used. Belladonna, for example, used to treat fever and conjunctivitis, caused fevers and inflamed eyes. When the subjects stopped taking the test medicine, their symptoms disappeared.

Having seen "symptoms" in healthy people, Dr. Hahnemann began thinking that these characteristic reactions were separate from disease, that symptoms were what the body did to combat illness, not the illness itself. This idea led to the primary tenet of homeopathy, what Hahnemann called the law of similars and what is popularly stated as "like cures like."

What is the law of similars?

Stated simply, the law maintains that a substance which causes an illness when taken in overdose by a healthy person, can stimulate the body to self-cure if it is taken in small doses by someone who is ill. Though controversial, this idea was not new in the eighteenth century. Hippocrates, the fourth-century Greek physician revered as the "Father of Medicine" said, "Through the like, disease is produced, and through the application of the like it is cured." Paracelsus, a fifteenth-century Swiss physician, wrote: ". . . bring together the same anatomy of the herbs and the same anatomy of the illness into one order. This simile gives you an understanding of the way in which you shall heal." Folk medicine holds that you treat a fever with heat—the medical application of the Native American sweat lodge. And twentieth-century medicine applies the principle under certain conditions: Allergy sufferers are given injections of the things they are allergic to; vaccinations introduce viruses so that the body can create antibodies to fight them; gold, which can cause joint pain, is used to relieve arthritis.

Hahnemann's contribution to this concept was his perception that symptoms are not the disease itself. As part of the disease process, symptoms represent the body's best efforts to combat the disease—what we now call the immune response—and any medicines that are used should be chosen for their power to assist the body's efforts. For example, mucus is one way that the body traps and expels pathogens (disease-causing microbes). When treating a cold or an allergy, a homeopath will suggest a remedy that enhances and accelerates mucus production, not a decongestant to abort it.

How is homeopathy different from regular medicine?

Where homeopathy and standard medicine, sometimes called allopathy, diverge is not point-by-point, but in the philosophy as a whole. Any treatment from a classic

homeopath will conform with all four of the main homeopathic principles—like cures like, minimal doses, single
medicines prepared according to homeopathic practice,
and prescribing based on an assessment of the totality
of symptoms. Treatments from allopathic doctors may
conform with some, but not with others. For example,
virtually all doctors agree that vaccinations are useful in
preventing the relevant viral infection, an example of
like curing like. But this treatment cannot be considered
homeopathic because the vaccines are not prepared in
accordance with homeopathic pharmaceutics, the vaccines may be mixed (as with DPT, the diphtheria-pertus-
sis-tetanus vaccine), and the vaccines are administered
prophylactically, that is, in the absence of symptoms.
Other points of difference arise from the preparation of
homeopathic remedies and from the standards for dosages.

How are the remedies made?

Homeopathic medicines are primarily derived from
plants, but some are made from minerals, such as calcium,
gold, iron, and various salts, or from certain animal products, such as bee or snake venom. There are more than
2,000 remedies derived from various sources.

Dr. Hahnemann wanted to find the smallest effective
doses of his medicines. He adamantly believed this would
allow for the greatest benefit with the least harm. Through
carefully monitored experiments, he evolved a systematic
practice of diluting and succussing (a form of agitating)
the materials for the remedies that reduced harmful effects
while increasing their potency. In homeopathy, this process of alternately diluting and succussing the solution is
called *potentizing*.

When working with plants, Dr. Hahnemann began by
making a mother tincture: He steeped the plant material

in water or alcohol to produce a concentrated solution. Then he diluted the tincture in specific ratios to create a range of strengths. When working with insoluble materials such as minerals, the substance was mixed with a milk sugar base and ground, or triturated, with a mortar and pestle. Here the various potencies were achieved by timing the grinding, placing the resulting paste in solution to make a tincture, then diluting it according to the established ratios.

These ratios persist today in the X-scale, C-scale, and M-scale remedy potencies. ("X" stands for 10, "C" for 100, and "M" for 1000.) In the X-scale, 1 drop of the mother tincture is diluted in 9 drops of pure water to make a 1X solution. Then one drop is taken from the 1X and added to 9 drops of pure water to make a 2X solution. One drop of 2X is added to 9 drops of water to make 3X, and so on. This process is repeated to create a range of strengths for the medicines. The same process is used to make C-scale and M-scale remedies, except in the C-scale the dilution ratio is 1 drop to 99 drops, and in the M-scale, it is 1 to 999.

The second part of the process seems a little mystical and is the source of much of the controversy surrounding homeopathy. Dilution was not sufficient to create effective remedies, extreme dilution, in fact, destroys the substance. Additional experimentation by Hahnemann revealed that agitating the solution by tapping the bottom of the vial against a moderately hard surface (such as a book) allowed the medicine to retain efficacy despite extreme dilution. This tapping is called *succussion* from a Latin word that means "to shake from beneath." Hahnemann discovered that the more he diluted and succussed, the stronger the remedy became; accordingly, he developed protocols for the number of succussions that should follow each dilution.

READING THE LABEL

The manufacture and distribution of homeopathic remedies is overseen by the FDA (Federal Drug Administra-
tion) and the HPUS (Homeopathic Pharmacopoeia of
the United States).

The remedy label includes the name of the remedy,
the potency (X-, C-, or M-scale), lot number, directions
for use, and some commonsense warnings, such as
"Keep Out of the Reach of Children."

The FDA requires an expiration date, which will be
stamped on the vial. Homeopathic remedies are reputed
to stay potent for decades, however. If you want to use
a remedy that has been stored for a long time, shake
the vial before taking the remedy. This informal succussion will restore the potency.

Under "indications" will be a list of up to 3 conditions for which the remedy can be used. Since there
simply isn't room on the vial to provide full details
about the remedy picture, consult the Materia Medica
later in this book or one of the classic texts (*see:* Bibliog-
raphy) for complete information about the individual
remedies.

Why does succussion increase the strength of the remedy?

In the *Organon of Medicine*, Hahnemann discussed the
presence of the "vital force," the spark that distinguishes
animate from inanimate matter. Someone in possession
of the vital force is alive; absent the vital force, one is
dead. Health is the vital force serenely at work; illness
is the vital force "deranged by . . . an agent inimical to
life." It is this force, this energy, that Hahnemann
believed is separated from the material substance by dilu-

tion, animated by succussion, and imprinted on the medium used for the remedy (usually milk sugar).

The vital force present in each substance has a unique pattern, and the pattern has a distinct curative property. Hahnemann compared it with magnetism: "The medicinal property of those material substances which we call medicines proper, relates only to their energy to call out alteration in the well-being of animal life. . . . Just as the nearness of a magnetic pole can communicate only magnetic energy to the steel (namely, by a kind of infection) but cannot communicate other properties (for instance, more hardness or ductility, etc.). And thus every special medicinal substance alters through a kind of infection, that well-being of man in a peculiar manner exclusively its own and not in a manner peculiar to another medicine, as certainly as the nearness of the child ill with small-pox will communicate to a healthy child only small-pox and not measles."

Contemporary practitioners make an analogy with sympathetic vibration: The string of an instrument keyed to a particular note will vibrate in the presence of that sound, even if it is not the source of that sound. So, too, will the vital force of one organism resonate with the analogous vital force of another to restore health. This vibration pattern is embedded in the remedy through the prescribed combination of dilution and succussion.

Which potencies are the strongest?

The homeopathic principle is that the more you dilute and succuss, the stronger the medicine becomes; therefore, the M-scale is the strongest, and the X-scale is the mildest. Within each scale, higher numbers indicate more dilutions; so, 12X is stronger than 6X, 200C is stronger than 30C, 2M is stronger than 1M.

How do I know which potency to use?

Another of the guiding principles of homeopathy is minimal dosing, that is, you should take the lowest possible dose the fewest number of times to restore your health. Hahnemann called this the "law of infinitesimals" and observed that a high potency, even of a correctly chosen remedy, can "prove injurious by its mere magnitude." He declined to give specific guidelines for dosages beyond recommending seeking the minutest amount and said that: "It is impossible . . . to tabulate in advance all imaginable cases. Pure experiment, careful observation of the sensitiveness of each patient and accurate experience can alone determine this *in each individual case.*" In other words, you are the best judge of how the remedy and your illness are interacting.

Some general guidelines have evolved over the decades that homeopathy has been in use. Use the following suggestions, beginning treatment with the lowest potency. As you become familiar with the remedies and the effects of different potencies, you will be better able to make effective selections. If necessary, the remedies can be taken more frequently to sustain their effects. X- and C-scale potencies are commonly available at health food stores and some pharmacies. M-scale remedies are used to address chronic conditions or entrenched, long-standing illnesses (whether mental or physical). Because their effects are so profound, M-scale remedies are not commonly available over the counter. They should be taken only under the supervision of an experienced homeopath.

The X-scale and lower potencies of the C-scale (12C) are helpful with people who are greatly debilitated or who are fragile even when they are healthy—young children and the elderly, for example. They are also helpful with illnesses and injuries such as skin rashes or muscle sprains that are considered external or superficial in homeopathic terms (*see box:* Planes of Illness). The X-scale and the midrange of the C-scale (30C) are appropriate for normally robust people with acute illnesses.

The higher ranges of the C-scale (200C and above) can be used in cases where there is a broad overlap between your symptoms and the remedy picture, or when acute symptoms are severe or incapacitating: high fever, frequent vomiting, intractable nasal mucus, pounding headache, for example.

PLANES OF ILLNESS

Illnesses can afflict any level of your being. Contemporary homeopaths use the following scale, published by George Vithoulkas in 1980, to assess the severity of an illness. The mental plane is the deepest level; the physical plane, the most superficial. There are degrees of depth within each plane as well. Knowing how deep the problem is helps you determine the potency of remedy. In general, the deeper the problem, the higher the potency of the appropriate remedy. Within each column, the conditions are listed in order from the deepest to the most superficial.

Physical	Emotional	Mental
Brain	Cuicidal depression	Confusion
Heart	Apathy	Delirium
Endocrine	Sadness	Paranoia
Liver	Anguish	Delusions
Lungs	Phobias	Lethargy
Kidneys	Anxiety	Dullness
Bone	Irritability	Lack of
Muscle	Dissatisfaction	Concentration
Skin		Forgetfulness
		Absentmindedness

What is a "remedy picture"?

In the course of proving a remedy, a variety of symptoms are elicited and cataloged. They are organized in the Materia Medica by the part of the body affected: mind, head, eyes, ears, nose, face, mouth, stomach, abdomen, stool, male/female, respiratory, heart, back, extremities, and skin. An additional category—called Modalities—addresses the things that make you feel better or worse, which may include eating or not eating, food cravings or aversions, weather conditions, sleep patterns, time of day or night.

This catalog of symptoms is the remedy picture. When selecting a remedy, you or your homeopath will review these descriptions, looking for the one that best matches the totality of your symptoms.

What is meant by "totality of symptoms"?

This idea is the fourth basic precept of homeopathy. When you become unwell, you develop a set of symptoms that reflect your body's fight to maintain its innate state of health. The symptoms are specific to the illness—a cold and a flu, for example, are similar yet distinct—but they are also specific to you, to the particular way that you manifest the illness. Homeopathy has always been a holistic system and takes all differences into account. Attention is given to the way an illness disrupts your mental and emotional health as well as your physical condition. For example, if you go to an allopathic doctor with a sore throat, you might not think to mention that your hands itch. This information is relevant to a homeopath and could be the difference between a remedy that helps and one that doesn't. While taking your case, a homeopath will ask questions designed to discover a broad range of symptoms. In self-care of acute illnesses, you would use the same process, just remember to choose remedies according to the immediate symptom picture, even in an ongoing illness. Continuing the previous example, if your sore throat persists, but your hands no longer itch, the soreness is part of the immediate symptom picture, but the itchiness is no longer a symptom and should not be considered when selecting a remedy.

Physical symptoms let you know whether you have a cold or the flu, a headache or a sinus infection, a pulled muscle or a broken bone. Other symptoms reveal your mental and emotional states—you want to be left alone or you want someone to bring you drinks and read you stories until you feel better. You may feel anxious or depressed, or perhaps normally you are quick-witted, but a cold makes you dull and forgetful.

When you are sick, you might seek particular environments because they help you feel better: You sit by an open window or turn on a fan because the moving air is soothing. Or you bundle up in blankets and lie still in the dark because that is soothing. You may also avoid things that make you feel worse; for example, you may be very hungry but refuse to eat because you can't keep anything down.

The weather or the time of day may influence how you feel. You might feel better in cool damp weather, worse in dry weather, and terrible if it's windy, no matter what the temperature or humidity. You may feel worse in the morning and better as the day goes on or just the opposite.

You may also manifest symptoms that seem contradictory; for example, you may have chills but crave cold drinks, or you may have a frequent, urgent desire to urinate, but urinating is painful and scanty. In homeopathy, these unexpected combinations are called *peculiars* and are often the most significant factors for determining an appropriate remedy.

The remedy pictures include a broad array of physical, mental, and emotional effects. Compare the array of symptoms you are experiencing to the effects described in the remedy profiles in the Materia Medica (Part Three). The remedy with greatest overlap with your condition is the one that will be the most help in relieving your illness.

Is a compound remedy more effective than a single remedy?

Dr. Hahnemann was opposed to using compound medicines. In the *Organon* he says: "In no case under treatment is it necessary and *therefore not permissible* to administer to a patient more than *one single simple medicinal* substance at a time." In accordance with this principle, classic homeopaths always look for the one remedy best suited to a particular case, and, as has been demonstrated, because each remedy influences a broad range of symptoms, a single well-chosen remedy will be effective over the range of those symptoms.

However, compound remedies can be helpful to the layman if you are having trouble identifying a remedy or in deciding between two or more. A compound medicine will broaden your chances of stumbling on one that works, but it may also result in so-called side effects— an inadvertent proving of the unnecessary medication.

How does a homeopath decide which remedy will be the most helpful?

Your homeopath will ask a lot of questions. This diagnostic interview may be short or quite long depending on whether your problem is acute or chronic, mild or severe, overt or subtle. An effective remedy for an acute condition can be recommended based primarily on the symptoms that are manifesting and a little information about how you cope with illness and who you are as a person. Remedies for serious or chronic conditions are determined after an extensive diagnostic interview. These recommendations are best made by an experienced (not merely trained) homeopath.

The questions will cover a wide range and some may seem wholly unrelated to the problem at hand. For example, a homeopath may ask about your sleep and eating habits, your energy level and emotional states, your mental acuity, and how the weather affects you. There will be questions about the specific character of the illness, for example: Does it start abruptly or come on slowly? Exactly what does it feel like? Are you better or worse at any particular time of day or night? After eating or not eating? Do you have any symptoms in addition to the primary problem—such as nausea or muscle pain with headache? Finally, there will be questions about your idiosyncratic reactions to your illness. Some people like to be left alone when they are ill, others prefer company. If you are chilly when sick, do you crave warmth or coolness? Is your appetite affected? Are you demanding or yielding, irritable or placid?

After the interview, the practitioner will consult two references: a Repertory and a Materia Medica. A Repertory is a dictionary of symptoms and illnesses with recommendations for treatment. The Materia Medica is a catalog of the remedies and their effects. The homeopath uses these books to *repertorize*, that is, match your particular array of symptoms to the remedy that resonates with the broadest number of them (*see*: "How to Use This Section" in Part Three, The Materia Medica).

When selecting a remedy to treat an acute illness, it

isn't necessary to match every symptom detailed in the remedy profile, or even a preponderance of them. In acute care, a remedy can help if it overlaps between 3 and 5 of your most pressing symptoms. In the case of chronic or severe illness, it is preferable to have a high degree of overlap between the remedy profile and the presenting symptoms. In all cases, the greater the overlap, the more effective the remedy.

If different symptoms come forward in the course of an acute illness, treat the symptoms as they arise. It is not unusual to use two or more remedies to address various symptoms throughout a cold, or to use different remedies to treat colds that arise at different times of the year (in homeopathy, a spring cold is different from a winter cold), or that affect different parts of the body in different sequences (a head-to-chest cold, for example, is different from a chest-to-head cold).

TAKING THE CASE

To determine which remedy will be helpful for self-care of an acute illness, ask yourself some or all of the following questions. Make a list of your responses and be as specific as possible with your answers. Compare your symptoms to those listed for the remedies in the Materia Medica (Part Three). The remedy that includes most of your symptoms, or most of your most troubling symptoms, will be the best choice for your particular condition.

1. How did the illness begin? Consider: left or right side, suddenly or gradually, after an injury, from eating or drinking, after exposure to weather.
2. Scan through your body. What symptoms, if any, are occurring in each area?
3. What are your most pressing symptoms?
4. If there is pain, what does it feel like? Where is it located?
5. If you have a cough, what is it like?
6. Do you have any discharges? If so, describe it (color, odor, consistency, benign or irritating).
7. Do you have a fever? Chills?
8. Are your bowels affected (constipation, diarrhea)?
9. Is your face pale or flushed? If flushed, what color is it (pink, red, purplish)? Are there dark circles under your eyes?
10. What makes you feel better? What makes you feel worse?
11. Is your appetite or thirst affected? Do you crave any foods or drinks? Are you averse to any foods or drinks?
12. Has your sleep pattern changed? How so?
13. Describe your mental state. Consider: ability to concentrate, patience level, alertness, forgetfulness.
14. Has your mood changed? What emotions do you feel most often and most powerfully?
15. Has your energy level changed?

Do I take homeopathic remedies like any other medicine?

Remedies come in several forms. All of them are available as lactose-based pellets (sometimes called globules), and some also come as a liquid (sometimes called a tincture). A few remedies—arnica and calendula, for example—are made as creams or gels and are applied topically like any other salve.

When taking pellets or liquids, place the remedy under your tongue. Avoid chewing or swallowing the pellets; you get better absorption if you let them dissolve in your mouth. (This takes a few minutes.)

One dose of a remedy is 1–3 pellets or 3 drops of a tincture. Doses are defined by time, not volume, that is, taking one pellet once is the same as taking a handful at once. You don't overdose on the remedy because it is a single dose. If, however, you take one pellet, then let 20 minutes elapse before taking another, you have taken two doses. Repeating doses over time increases the effects of the remedy.

When dispensing pellets, avoid handling them. Tap them into the cap or onto a piece of paper, then pick up only as many as you need. Pour any extras back into the vial. Handling the pellets can contaminate them. If you put contaminated pellets into the vial, they can alter the entire contents.

When taking homeopathic remedies in any form, avoid strong-smelling substances—mint (toothpaste, food, candies, teas), camphor, or menthol (used in cold remedies and cosmetics)—for 20 to 30 minutes before and after a dose. You should also avoid drinking coffee, black tea, or cola and eating or drinking chocolate for the same amount of time. These substances can negate the effect of the remedy.

Store the remedies in a cool, dry place (not the frequently hot and steamy bathroom medicine cabinet). Keep them away from strongly aromatic items, such as perfumes and cosmetics, and any preparations that contain mint, menthol, or camphor.

How often should I take the remedy?

Take the remedies on an as-needed basis, not by a clock-based schedule. Take one dose and wait until you notice an improvement. Do not repeat the dose as long as the improvement continues. When the improvement levels off or subsides, take another dose. The cycle of improvement may be long or short—as short as 10 or 15 minutes—but as long as improvement is under way, additional medication is not needed.

How do I know it's working?

After taking a remedy, one of three things will happen: You will feel better; you will feel worse; or you will feel the same. The reactions depend on whether you have taken a well-chosen remedy.

If you take an appropriate remedy, you will begin to feel better almost immediately. You may feel better mentally or spiritually—more hopeful, for example—before you feel better physically, but feeling better on any level is a sign that the remedy is appropriate to the condition and is working. (If you have taken an appropriate remedy, especially if it is a relatively high potency, you may very quickly fall asleep. When you wake up, you will be greatly improved.)

Another sign that a remedy is working is feeling worse. Remember that homeopathy distinguishes between symptoms and illness, putting symptoms on the side of health.

If the symptoms you already have accelerate—a situation that homeopaths call an aggravation—consider it a sign of improvement. Your body's natural defense mechanisms have been strengthened and are fighting the illness. An aggravation, sometimes called a healing crisis, usually passes quickly (within 2 to 3 hours), and then you will begin to feel better. An aggravation is usually caused by taking too high a potency. If you get an aggravation, switch to a lower potency of the remedy or take it less frequently.

You can have both reactions at once: believing that you are getting better even though your symptoms are aggravated. This seeming contradiction is an example of Hering's laws of cure (*see box*: Hering's Laws of Cure), feeling better at a deep level (your mental or spiritual self) while feeling worse closer to the surface (your physical symptoms) is also a sign of improvement.

If, however, you take an inappropriate remedy, you will also feel worse, or no better on any level. The difference here is that none of your symptoms abate within 2 hours of taking the remedy. If this happens, try another remedy.

Stay with one remedy for as long as it helps. Change to another remedy only if the first one is ineffective, or if it stops creating improvement.

HERING'S LAWS OF CURE

Dr. Constantine Hering (1800–1880), a German physician who is considered the father of American homeopathy, observed that illness resolves in predictable stages. In the mid-1800s, he codified these observations into three principles that are used to gauge the general progress of healing.

1. Symptoms resolve in the reverse order from which they appeared.
2. Symptoms resolve from top to bottom (head to feet).
3. Symptoms resolve in more important organs first, followed by less important organs.

Are there any side effects?

It is not entirely true that homeopathy has no side effects. Homeopathy arose through a series of clinical trials, or *provings,* in which symptoms of illnesses were deliberately created in healthy people. If you choose an inappropriate remedy, you may find yourself doing a proving, that is, you may develop symptoms that the remedy is capable of eliciting in addition to the symptoms you already have. The symptoms generated in a proving are transient, but they are real and may be uncomfortable while they are manifesting.

Over and above that, however, Hahnemann rejected the idea that you can acknowledge some effects of a remedy and dismiss others. An assessment of the totality of symptoms is a cornerstone of homeopathic philosophy, and so all effects, even those that another treatment system might discount as ''side'' effects, are accepted as part of the remedy picture and acknowledged as desirable in some cases.

Can I use homeopathy if I am taking other medicines?

Dr. Hahnemann was opposed to mixing therapies. However, the standard medical practices in place in his lifetime included radical and harmful procedures such as blood-letting, purging, and fasting, and medicines derived from toxic chemicals such as arsenic and mercury.

Contemporary practitioners are more lenient. Combining therapies can be very effective, with a few caveats. Be sure you have proper supervision from trained and experienced people. Stay alert to your condition and keep everyone informed of your progress. Avoid combining so many practices that it becomes difficult to sort out what is useful. Drop practices that do not help and, especially, drop ones that are harmful.

Whether used alone or as a complement to standard medical treatments, homeopathy can speed healing—safely, rapidly, deeply, gently, and effectively in a wide variety of illnesses and injuries.

PART TWO

HEADACHE

FREQUENTLY ASKED QUESTIONS

Why does my head hurt?

All pain is nerve pain. It occurs when the nerve is stimulated, usually by pressure from the surrounding tissues. The pressure may be due to muscle contraction, inflammation, or bloating. For example, in a tension headache the muscles are held in a continuous state of contraction. This state creates pressure on the nerves embedded in the muscle fibers, and the stimulated nerves send signals to the brain that are interpreted as pain. In a vascular headache, such as migraine, the blood vessels usually dilate (expand), causing pressure on the nerves in the vessel walls. As with the muscle contraction headache, the pressure is perceived as pain. The brain is alerted to this change with pain signals. Sinus headache is similar in that the swelling and impaction of the sinuses causes pressure on the nerve fibers, and the pressure is perceived as pain.

Are headaches a symptom of an underlying illness?

Although it may be frequent, severe, and debilitating, most headache pain is not a symptom of another illness. Fewer than 10 percent of the people who consult doctors for headache have a separate illness. However, headache is a symptom of a variety of ailments, including arthritis, hypertension, and eye disease, so do read through the conditions described in "When to See a Doctor" to determine whether you need to be tested and treated for another condition.

Most often, though, the pain of a headache *is* the illness. Its triggers are subtle and persistent and—as anyone with chronic headache pain will tell you—difficult to treat. The pain signals from your nerves to your brain are physiological calls for action. The nerves are saying "There's a problem here. Fix it." In an ideal situation the brain does. In response to this cry for help, the brain deploys a cascade of biochemicals to reverse the problem. But sometimes the body needs more help than it can get on its own and the goal of homeopathy is to enhance, rather than disrupt, the body's own defenses.

WHEN TO SEE A DOCTOR

Headache is rarely a symptom of a serious underlying illness. Fewer than 10 percent of the people who seek medical help for their headaches have anything other than headache (and fewer than 1 percent have brain tumors). There are, however, many situations when you should have your headaches evaluated by a doctor. In general, the guiding factors are *onset, persistence and frequency,* and *severity.* You should see a doctor if you experience some or all of the following symptoms.

See a Doctor If . . .

Onset

. . . the pain is new, i.e., unlike your usual headache, or you have rarely or never had headaches before
. . . the pain is sudden, intense, and unbearable
. . . you get your first headache in your 40s or 50s
. . . the headache comes from exertion (coughing, laughing, or sneezing, lifting or straining, bending over, exercise, sex)
. . . you awaken in the night from the pain

Persistence and Frequency

. . . headaches become more frequent
. . . you get headaches more than three times a week
. . . the headaches increase in frequency or become continuous
. . . you take over-the-counter medications on a daily basis to prevent or relieve your headaches
. . . the headache does not respond to treatment

Severity

. . . the pain increases in severity over weeks or months
. . . you have debilitating pain that interferes with your ability to lead a normal life

---

SEE A DOCTOR IMMEDIATELY IF ...

... you get a headache after an injury, especially to the head, neck, or back

... you also have eye or ear pain or symptoms such as a discharge from the eyes or ears, ringing in the ears

... you experience other symptoms with the headache, especially: flu symptoms (fever, sore throat, nausea, joint pain or stiffness), neurological disturbances (slurred speech, blurred or double vision, coordination or balance problems, fainting, seizures or convulsions, numbness or tingling), drowsiness, weakness, disorientation or confusion

---

Why doesn't my doctor understand how much this hurts?

Your doctor does understand that you hurt. But because pain perception has emotional as well as physical components, it cannot be measured in absolute terms the same way that, for example, the stages of healing for a broken bone can be measured. Pain is always relative and its perception depends on two factors: *pain threshold* and *pain tolerance*.

Pain threshold is simply the level of stimulus—how much pressure—that is needed for the sensation to be felt and interpreted as pain. This threshold may be reflexive and almost instantaneous, as when you jerk your hand away from a hot surface or leap back from a loud noise, or it may be gradual, as when pain from an infected tooth grows and grows.

Pain tolerance, on the other hand, is a term for the idiosyncratic way each of us interprets the sensation and severity of pain. This perception varies from person to person and, oftentimes, within the same person. Some people can rest relatively contentedly after major surgery and never want pain medication; others are so debilitated by any pain that they need an anesthetic to have a splinter removed.

Since the perception of pain is so idiosyncratic, it can be more perplexing than illuminating in medical philosophies that look for universal standards and solutions.

How is the approach to diagnosis different in homeopathy?

A homeopath will be very interested in how you perceive and describe the pain you experience. A crushing pain (pressing inward) is significantly different from one that is bursting (pressing out). A pain on the left side takes a different remedy from one on the right side. Pain that starts on the left and moves to the right is different from one that is localized. Time and weather are also important. Night pain is different from day pain. Pain brought on by or worsened by cold, heat, humidity, or wind is treated differently from pains that are relieved or eradicated by those conditions.

When you consult a homeopath, she will ask you a series of very detailed questions about yourself, your life and habits, and your ailment. (This diagnostic interview is called *taking the case*.) Many of the questions will be the same or similar to those that a doctor would ask: When did the pain start? How long does it last? Are you taking anything for it? Is it helping? Is the pain generalized or localized? Have you noticed whether it starts after you eat certain foods?

In addition to these kinds of questions, a homeopath will you ask about your mental and emotional state—both when you are in the throes of a headache and when you are not. She may ask: Are you alert or forgetful? Do

your moods shift or are they stable? Do you want to be
left alone when you don't feel well or do you prefer
company? Additional questions will cover your eating
habits; sleep and dream patterns; and your level of con-
tentment with your job, your family, and your social life.

It is best not to try to outguess the therapist. In order
to recommend an effective homeopathic remedy, the therapist must have accurate information. It is not in your
best interest to claim that you are sensitive, laugh and
cry easily, and feel better walking outdoors in a light
breeze when in fact you prefer to be indoors, would rather
die than cry, and tend to be sarcastic. However much you
may wish that you fit a particular description or believe
that it is more desirable to be a certain way, misinforma-
tion will lead to misdiagnosis. There are no wrong
answers in the quest for health.

What can I do to combat headaches?

First, have some basic checkups: see your internist or an
ENT (ear, nose, and throat) specialist, have your eyes
and vision tested, and go to the dentist. Many transient
headaches are caused by eyestrain from an incorrect eye-
glass prescription, dental problems, poor jaw alignment,
poor head and neck posture, or structural abnormalities
in the nasal sinuses (such as polyps or a deviated septum)
that contribute to blockage and infection.

Keep a record of your headaches (*see*: Using the Headache Diary) and try to identify whether there are patterns
of onset that you can change or avoid. Your headache
might be triggered by the residue of a cleaning product
used in your office or by caffeine withdrawal on the
weekend. A food allergy may trigger a headache. Frequent alternations of hot and cold environments, such as
going in and out of heated buildings in winter or cooled

ones in summer, may give you a headache. Do what you can to change your habits or your interaction with the environment.

Examine your family's medical history. Particular kinds of headaches tend to run in families, migraine, for instance, and cluster headaches. You can't change a genetic predisposition to an illness, but the information is helpful in diagnosis and treatment.

Is a medical diagnosis helpful to a homeopath?

Any information you have about your condition is helpful. Hundreds of remedies have been developed over the decades since homeopathy began. Each remedy fits a particular constellation of symptoms and many of the remedy profiles are long and detailed. A medical diagnosis, such as migraine or cluster headache, coupled with the specific information you provide about your particular condition, will help your homeopath identify an appropriate remedy more quickly.

How are headaches categorized?

Headaches fall into three basic categories—*tension* (or *muscle contraction*), *vascular,* or *pathological*—according to their physiology and symptoms. A subcategory of headache, *mixed* headache, has recently been identified. Mixed headaches exhibit symptoms of both tension and vascular headaches. This discovery has led some researchers to question whether tension headaches and vascular headaches, in particular migraine, are distinct illnesses in fact or simply manifestations of a single underlying neurological disorder. Further investigation is being done to examine this theory.

Tension, or *muscle contraction,* headaches arise due to changes brought on by holding the muscles of your face, head, neck, and back in a state of contraction. The contraction reduces blood flow, inhibiting the delivery of oxygen and the release of lactic acid and other waste products which causes the sensation of stiff and sore muscles.

Vascular headaches are related to changes in the diameter of your blood vessels. The vessels may constrict or dilate, or first do one then the other, but in either case, the result is a throbbing, pulsating pain in the head. Migraine and cluster headaches are in this category.

Pathological headaches are those that arise due to an existing pathology, or illness, such as hypertension, arthritis, or sinusitis. Since pain is a deviation from the normal state, premenstrual headaches are included in this category.

How can I tell what kind of headache I have?

The symptoms of the various headaches are fairly distinct, so reading through the descriptions given in the next section will help you classify your headache. No book can substitute for a clinical diagnosis, however; so, after using the headache diary to track and analyze your symptoms, do talk with your doctor. It is especially important to identify and treat or to rule out any underlying conditions for which headache may be a symptom, not the disease. (*See*: When to See A Doctor.)

Are there medical tests to diagnose headaches?

Headaches are commonly diagnosed by symptoms. Simple tests—such as a physical, a dental checkup, or an eye exam—combined with a clear description of the symptoms and pattern of your headaches are usually all that are needed for a diagnosis. If these tests fail to identify the problem, additional tests, such as X rays, a CAT scan, or an MRI may be undertaken to find out whether another condition is causing or aggravating the headache.

X rays. Less accurate than other imaging techniques because the density of the body tends to create shadows in the image, X rays are still helpful in diagnosing bone diseases, such as arthritis, as well as sinus infections and fractures.

CAT scan. Sometimes called a CT scan, CAT scans are similar to X rays, except that the area being examined is smaller. CAT is the acronym for *computerized axial tomography*. ''Tomography'' is radiography (X-raying) without shadows. ''Axial'' refers to the narrow cross-sections that are taken from a particular axis, or direction, and ''computerized'' means that a computer is part of the equipment.

During a CAT scan, a narrow X ray beam takes a picture of a cross-section of your head and maps the bones, muscles, organs, tissues, and fluids. The technician may take about a dozen of these pictures, each one taking one or two seconds to complete. The images are fed into a computer that translates them into black, white, and gray tones and prints them out. Your doctor will analyze the images for abnormalities that suggest disease. CAT scans are helpful in identifying head injuries, blood clots, sinus infections, brain diseases, and aneurysms (dilated blood vessels that are associated with stroke).

MRI. This imaging system uses a magnetic field rather

than radiation to generate pictures of the body's soft tissues. The test itself is painless, but some people find the environment of the test unsettling. The machine makes a noise similar to a jackhammer (although not as loud), and you must lie still in a tube not much larger than your body, a situation some people find claustrophobic. The test usually lasts for about 45 minutes. An MRI will aid the diagnosis of a tumor, hydrocephalus, sinusitis, aneurysm, TMJ (temporomandibular joint problems), and spinal cord disease.

What if my headaches don't fall into one the main categories?

Any headache that occurs after an injury, especially an injury to the head, neck, or back should be considered a medical emergency. The side effects of head trauma can be crippling or fatal. It is better to be a little embarrassed about overreacting than risk the possible consequences from an undiagnosed injury.

Absent an injury, if your headaches are not persistent or severe and if they don't have any particular pattern, such as a weekday/weekend pattern, it is likely that their cause is in your environment or is the result of some behavior that can be tracked and changed. Any number of things can trigger headache. Food allergies, food sensitivities (not a full-blown allergy), and hunger are common causes. (For a list of foods that have been implicated in triggering headache, *see*: The Migraine Diet.) You may have environmental triggers—some people are susceptible to headache when the seasons or the weather changes. Certain odors—a cleaner that contains ammonia, for example—may give you a headache. An allergy to dust or pollen can provoke a headache.

A common "other" headache is the rebound headache. Typically, these headaches occur in people who drink a lot of coffee at work and not so much on the weekend. Caffeine has a profound effect on the state of your blood vessels, so much so that it is sometimes prescribed as a migraine medication. The weekend withdrawal from caffeine frequently results in an intense, throbbing, migraine-like headache. Another rebound headache example is seen in people who use over-the-counter medications daily in an effort to prevent headaches. If they skip a dose, they get a headache. This response reinforces the notion that persistent use of the medicine wards off the pain, but in fact it is the abuse of the medication and subsequent derangement of the body's normal state that causes the headache.

Using the headache diary is particularly helpful for identifying the causes of transient headaches. Record the circumstances that surround your headaches, especially if they occur only every month or so. The diary will help you to identify things that could easily be forgotten—eating a second or third hot dog, for example—but that may be causing the pain.

DEFINING HEADACHE

TENSION, OR MUSCLE CONTRACTION, HEADACHES

These headaches, are the most common and account for 75 to 90 percent of headaches for which people seek treatment. Unlike migraine, which afflicts women more than men or cluster headaches which men suffer with more than women, tension headaches affect men and women about equally.

Tension Headaches

The "tension" in a tension headache refers to holding the muscles of your head, face, and neck in contraction. This contraction reduces blood flow, encourages the retention of lactic acid and other waste products, and exerts pressure on nerve fibers—all of which can cause pain. Although the headache may arise during a period of stress—as when working toward a fast-approaching deadline—it may just as easily result from remaining in one position for an extended period of time—while studying, writing or typing, or playing cards, for example.

The headache may be acute (temporary) or chronic. Chronic tension headaches occur frequently, at least twice a week, and may persist for up to a week. Usually a sufferer will wake with a headache or the headache starts early in the day. Chronic tension headaches may be related to depression or other psychological difficulties.

Whether acute or chronic, typically the pain is not incapacitating and you can work through the discomfort without aggravating the pain. The symptoms are usually limited to head pain—there is no nausea or visual disturbances, as with migraine—and the headaches usually respond to treatment with over-the-counter medicines, naps, relaxation techniques, breaks from sedentary work, mild physical exercise, or simply a release from the stressful situation.

If you suffer with tension headaches, your diary entries will include some or all of these symptoms:

Onset: Gradual, usually in the morning. With deadline pressure. From remaining in one position for too long.

Location: Bilateral pain, either both sides (temples) or forehead and base of skull.

Sensation: Viselike pain, generalized, dull steady ache; does not throb or pound.

Modalities

Worse: In the morning (wake with pain or pain starts in the morning).

Better: From sleep, relaxation, change of position, release from tense situation.

Concomitants: Neck and shoulder pain, stiffness, may affect shoulders and arms.

Mentals and Generals: Depressed, anxious, feeling overwhelmed.

Homeopathic remedies that may be helpful for tension headaches include:

Aconitum napellus, Apis mellifica, Calcarea carbonica, Colocynthis, Ignatia, Iris versicolor, Magnesia phosphorica, Natrum muriaticum, Spigelia

Eyestrain

Except in cases of astigmatism, headaches attributed to eyestrain are more likely to be tension headaches that arise from contracting the muscles in the face, head, and neck. An eyestrain headache may also be sinus-related.

If you get headaches after driving long distances, reading, sewing, or doing close craft work, have an eye exam. If you are not astigmatic and the prescription for your glasses (if any) is correct, taking deliberate and regular breaks from the work and moving around a bit should prevent the headache. Warm or cold applications often provide relief. If these simple measures don't help or if the headaches persist despite at-home treatment, see your doctor to rule out sinus problems.

If you suffer from eyestrain, your diary entries will be very similar to those for tension headaches. The main exception will be the location. The dull ache of eyestrain centers around the eyes and eye sockets, forehead, and cheekbones. Your eyes will feel hot and tired and may be red and inflamed. These headaches can be distinguished from sinus-related headaches by persistence, severity of the pain, and, possibly, by a seasonal onset. Sinus headache is usually more painful and persistent than eyestrain.

Homeopathic remedies that may be helpful for eyestrain include:

Argentum nitricum, Gelsemium, Natrum muriaticum, Ruta graveolens

TMJ (Temporomandibular Joint Syndrome)
TMJ is defined by moderate or severe pain in and around the joint between the temples and the jaw (or *mandible*). The pain may extend to the ear, and tinnitus (ringing or buzzing in the ears) or deafness may accompany it. The pain is worse when chewing and the joint may click or pop when chewing, talking, or yawning.

The condition may arise due to stress and tension, ill-fitting dentures, poor alignment of the jaw or teeth, or an illness such as rheumatoid arthritis. Stress-related symptoms include clenching the jaw or grinding the teeth. These actions often occur while sleeping and are, therefore, difficult to control. See your dentist and doctor to determine what is causing the pain. Stress reduction and a simple exercise program to correct your posture will help relieve the problem.

Homeopathic remedies that may be helpful for TMJ include:

Calcarea carbonica, Lachesis, Sanguinaria

Exertion Headaches
Headaches that erupt after physical exertion—regardless of whether the exertion is strenuous, such as running, or mild, such as coughing or laughing—must be evaluated by a doctor. This is one of the relatively rare situations when headache may be a symptom of a severe illness. In about 10 percent of the cases involving exertion headaches, a brain tumor or aneurysm is the cause.

After ruling out any underlying illnesses, consider treating exertion headaches with exercise to improve your stamina and general health.

Homeopathic remedies that may be helpful for exertion headaches include:

Aconitum napellus, Argentum nitricum, Arnica, Belladonna, Bryonia, Calcarea carbonica, Ferrum phosphoricum, Iris versicolor, Natrum muriaticum, Nux vomica (especially if related to sexual activity), Sulphur

VASCULAR HEADACHES

Changes in the diameter of your blood vessels, either dilation or constriction, can cause headache pain. Migraine and cluster headaches are the two most prevalent examples, but people who have hypertension and anyone who overindulges in alcohol may also get a vascular headache.

Migraine

The word "migraine" is derived from a Greek word, *hemicrania*, that means "half the head." Classic migraine pain occurs on one side of the head, centering around the eye or temple, and may be accompanied by numbness, tingling, or weakness down the body on the same side.

Migraine afflicts women more than men, with women accounting for about 75 percent of migraineurs, as its sufferers are sometimes called. Susceptibility to migraines runs in families and migraines may triggered by a range of factors from stress to processed foods (*see*: The Migraine Diet). The pain usually occurs in two phases—vasoconstriction followed by vasodilation; each phase has a specific array of symptoms. During vasoconstriction, reduced blood flow causes tingling or prickling sensations, visual disturbances (aura, hallucination), and disrupted perceptions of heat and cold. The subsequent dilation causes the throbbing, pounding, pulsating pain.

Migraines typically have symptoms beyond head pain,

including nausea and/or vomiting, dizziness, numbness. While the headache is in force, you may be hypersensitive to light (especially sunlight), noise, odors, touch—the slightest stimulation of any of your senses can exacerbate the headache.

If you suffer with migraine, your diary entries will include some or all of these symptoms:

Onset: When the pain hits, it hits suddenly, but typically it is preceded by a procession of warning symptoms that may include mood changes, changes in energy levels, heightened sensory perception, food cravings (especially for candy or cake), excessive yawning, and speech or memory problems.

Within an hour of the pain's onset, a small percentage of migraine sufferers experience visual disturbances such as aura (flashing lights, shimmering zigzag lines, black spots) or diminished vision, and numbness or tingling in lips or hands. In rare cases, the disturbance is so profound that the person may hallucinate, suffer temporary blindness, or be unable to speak.

Location: Pain on one side of the head, or localized in one spot. During the headache the pain may switch from one side to the other or gradually envelop the whole head.

Sensation: Intense throbbing, pulsating pain. Pain that is constant and disabling.

Modalities

Worse: With movement (especially bending over or leaning forward). Light, noise, aromas, breezes.

Better: Lying still in a dark quiet room. Pain may be relieved by vomiting.

Concomitants: Nausea and vomiting. Neck or shoulder pain, numbness in the extremities. Impaired coordination. Dizziness. Diarrhea or increased urination. In extreme cases, you may experience weakness on one side of the body, or tingling through the face, lips, tongue, or fingers on the painful side. Speech or memory impairment.

Mentals and Generals: The person must go to bed in a still, dark, quiet room and wait it out. Aversion to eating or drinking; even water may be vomited. When the headache ends, you may feel a burst of energy and hunger or feel completely drained and exhausted. Your muscles may feel bruised and stiff as from overexertion. The exhaustion may persist for a day or so. Your emotions may be unstable, with mood shifts from depression to euphoria.

Homeopathic remedies that may be helpful for migraine include:

Argentum nitricum, Arsenicum album, Belladonna, Bryonia, Calcarea carbonica, China officinalis, Colocynthis, Gelsemium, Ignatia, Iris versicolor, Kali bichromicum, Lachesis, Natrum muriaticum, Nux vomica, Pulsatilla, Sanguinaria, Spigelia

For left-sided pain: Argentum nitricum, Bryonia, Natrum muriaticum, Nux vomica, Spigelia

For right-sided pain: Belladonna, Iris versicolor, Kali bichromicum, Sanguinaria

For headache with gastrointestinal disturbances (including nausea or vomiting): Argentum nitricum, Arsenicum album, Bryonia, Gelsemium, Iris versicolor, Natrum muriaticum, Nux vomica, Pulsatilla, Sanguinaria

For headache with visual disturbances: Belladonna, Gelsemium, Ignatia, Iris versicolor, Kali bichromicum, Natrum muriaticum, Nux vomica, Sanguinaria

THE MIGRAINE DIET

A variety of foods have been implicated as migraine triggers. If you include these foods in your diet, try limiting or eliminating them and see if it reduces the frequency or intensity of your headaches.

Dairy products
Buttermilk
Cheddar, Gruyere, Brie, and other ripened cheeses
Sour cream
Chocolate milk
Yogurt

Meat and Fish
Cured, smoked, or processed meats and fish, such as bacon, bratwurst, beef jerky, corned beef, hot dogs or corn dogs, pepperoni, pork and beans, Spam, sausage, smoked fish, pickled herring
Lunch meats, including those made with turkey, such as bologna, ham, liverwurst, pastrami, salami
Fresh meats such as chicken livers, pork

Fruits and vegetables
Avocados, bananas, beans (garbanzo, lima, navy, pinto), citrus fruits (grapefruit, oranges) and their juice, nuts and nut butters, onions, papayas, pea pods, raisins, sauerkraut, seeds (pumpkin, sesame, sunflower)

Yeast breads and cake, including raised doughnuts

Beverages
Alcohol (especially beer, bourbon, red wine, and sherry), coffee, tea, chocolate, caffeinated sodas

Condiments
MSG (Chinese foods, canned and processed foods), soy sauce, vinegar

Pickled foods

Cluster Headaches
Cluster headaches have the dubious distinction of being the most painful headache possible. They affect less than 1 percent of the population, and 90 percent of that 1 percent are men. Many of the people afflicted are heavy smokers, and, typically, their first attacks come in their 20s or 30s. Unlike migraine, cluster headaches generally do not run in families. Because they are rare and transient, albeit intense, cluster headaches are frequently misdiagnosed as sinusitis, dental trouble, or an allergic reaction.

The pain comes in bouts, or clusters, of recurring headaches. The pain may be short-lived, as short as 15 minutes or as long as 3 hours, but the headaches will recur several times a day, at approximately the same time every day, for up to 16 weeks. Cluster headaches seem to be an all-or-nothing proposition: You may be headache-free and headache-resistant for months or years, then when another cycle occurs, be hypersensitive to triggers.

The pain of a cluster headache is excruciating. It does not throb or pulsate as with migraine, but rather builds in a steady crescendo, then subsides. It is tightly defined in one temple or behind one eye. At its peak, you may pace, rock, scream, or bang your head against a wall, desperate for relief. The pain is so bad and the anxiety over anticipating the pain during headache-free periods can be so intense that a sufferer may consider suicide.

If you suffer with cluster headaches, your diary entries will include some or all of these symptoms:
  Onset: Sudden, no preliminary symptoms. Cyclic: recurring at the same time of day or at regular intervals, for example 12 hours apart. Triggers may include alcohol, hot or cold wind blowing in the face, seasonal changes, or time shifts, as from standard time to daylight saving time.

Location: Tightly circumscribed pain, one side of the head, one spot on the head, or behind one eye.

Sensation: An excruciating, searing, boring pain, "as if a hot poker was thrust in the eye." The pain builds steadily, peaks, then subsides. The pain may radiate through the face to the jaw, teeth, temple, nose, or chin.

Concomitants: Nose may become congested or runny on the painful side. The eye on the painful side may become red, bloodshot, and teary; the lid may droop. The face may flush red or pink.

Mentals and Generals: Cannot sit still because the pain is so intense; seeks relief in motion: restless pacing, head-banging, rocking. The person will be agitated, desperate for relief (some have injured themselves in their efforts to stop the pain), and, in extreme cases, suicidal.

Homeopathic remedies that may be helpful for cluster headaches include:

Aconitum napellus, Argentum nitricum, Belladonna, Bryonia, China officinalis, Ignatia, Lachesis, Nux vomica, Ruta graveolens, Sanguinaria, Spigelia

For left-sided pain: Argentum nitricum, Bryonia, Nux vomica, Spigelia

For right-sided pain: Belladonna, Sanguinaria

Aurum metallicum (metallic gold), a remedy not detailed in the Materia Medica in this book because of its limited use in other kinds of headache, may be particularly helpful for cluster headache. If your headaches are marked by pain so violent and unbearable that it provokes profound despair and thoughts of suicide, try Aurum. Other symptoms that indicate Aurum are extreme sensitivity to light, facial pain (especially in and around the eyes, nose, and jaw), sinus congestion or discharge, restlessness, an intense drive to hurry (cannot do things fast enough), and insomnia—but its outstanding characteristic is suicidal depression.

Hangover

Overconsumption of alcohol causes vessel dilation which can result in the same kind of blinding, pounding, sick headache and acute nausea that defines migraine. Your individual tolerance will determine how much is too much; for some people, one or two drinks can be enough to cause a hangover. Also, some spirits—sherry, beer, and red wine, for example—are more likely to induce a hangover than others.

The best cure, of course, is prevention—don't drink yourself sick. If it's too late for that, drinking caffeinated beverages may help to tighten up the blood vessels and ice packs will relieve the pain. Whatever you do, don't try the hair of the dog. More alcohol will only make the problem worse.

If you get a hangover headache, you will have some or all of these symptoms:

Onset: After overconsumption of alcohol, rich food, stimulants. Wakes with pain.

Location: Temples or generalized.

Sensation: Throbbing, pounding, pulsating.

Modalities

    Worse: In the morning. With movement.

    Better: Staying still. Cold drinks (nonalcoholic) and applications.

Concomitants: Nausea, fatigue, lightheaded or dizzy, pallor, dehydration, trembling.

Homeopathic remedies that may be helpful for hangover headaches include:

Arsenicum album, Nux vomica, Ruta graveolens, Sanguinaria

MIXED HEADACHES

Headache researchers have identified a headache pattern that combines symptoms of tension headache and migraine. These so-called mixed headaches have led some specialists to believe that chronic tension headache and migraine are not separate illnesses but rather the two poles of a continuum of one illness. Because chronic tension headache and migraine can interfere with sleep and are associated with depression, they may be the result of disrupted or inadequate serotonin metabolism. (Serotonin is a brain chemical that controls sleep, the sensation of dull pain, emotions, and the sense of well-being. Abnormal serotonin metabolism also contributes to depression.)

Mixed headaches typically begin when you are in your 30s or 40s, are accompanied by depression, sleep disturbances, or anxiety, and afflict people who have a personal or family history of depression, alcoholism and/or substance abuse—including overuse of analgesics such as aspirin. The modalities and mentals and generals will be the same as those for migraine and tension headaches.

If you suffer with mixed headaches, your diary entries will include some or all of these symptoms:

Onset: From tightening muscles to holding head still (usually during a migraine).

Location: Generalized.

Sensation: Constant headache. Steady, squeezing, band-like pain.

Concomitants: Nausea, vomiting. Hypersensitivity to light. Changes in blood vessels.

Homeopathic remedies that may be helpful for mixed headaches include:

>Aconitum napellus, Apis mellifica, Argentum nitricum, Arsenicum album, Belladonna, Bryonia, Calcarea carbonica, Colocynthis, Gelsemium, Ignatia, Iris versicolor, Kali bichromicum, Lachesis, Natrum muriaticum, Nux vomica, Pulsatilla, Sanguinaria, Spigelia, Sulphur

REBOUND HEADACHES

Sometimes called withdrawal headaches, these occur when you reduce the amount of a substance, typically caffeine or, ironically, over-the-counter headache or sinus medications, that you consume. The so-called "weekend migraine" is usually not a true migraine but a rebound headache with migraine-like symptoms caused by reduced intake of caffeine. Similarly, daily doses of over-the-counter drugs may contribute to the daily onset of headaches rather than relieving them.

If your diary suggests that you are having rebound headaches, avoid the temptation to go cold turkey. Wean yourself from the substance by gradually and consistently reducing your intake over a period of two to four weeks. Talk with your doctor as well as your homeopath to devise an effective plan to manage your health while you are withdrawing, and your headaches after you are clean. Medical supervision is especially important if you have become dependent on analgesics since your blood pressure may be affected.

Caffeine Withdrawal Headaches

Although generally considered benign, caffeine actually has a powerful effect on your body. It constricts your blood vessels, prevents the re-absorption of adrenaline (which is why you're so very alert), and disrupts sleep.

Any of these factors can trigger a headache in someone susceptible to headaches, but the main problem arises when someone habituated to a certain level of caffeine misses a "dose" or skips it altogether. In this case, the blood vessels dilate and a throbbing, migraine-like headache erupts. If you drink a lot of coffee, tea, or carbonated sodas (especially colas), monitor your intake in conjunction with your headaches. Similarly, if you take pain relievers that contain caffeine (*see*: Caffeine and Pain Relievers) be aware that you may be perpetuating the root problem rather than correcting it.

Note: If you are susceptible to caffeine headaches and your caffeine source is coffee, cutting down or switching to decaf may not be enough. Coffee contains several chemicals that produce physiological effects similar to caffeine. These chemicals are not processed out when coffee is decaffeinated. You may have to give up coffee entirely.

If you suffer with caffeine withdrawal headaches, your diary entries will include some or all of these symptoms:

Onset: Cyclic, typically occur only on weekends or vacations. Wakes with pain.

Location: Generalized.

Sensation: Throbbing, pounding, "sick" headache.

Modalities

Worse: In the morning.

Better: Resuming caffeine intake.

Concomitants: Pallor, trembling, nausea.

Mentals and Generals: Lassitude. Irritable, short-tempered if disturbed.

Homeopathic remedies that may be helpful for caffeine withdrawal headaches include:

Bryonia, Gelsemium, Ignatia, Iris versicolor, Lachesis, Natrum muriaticum, Nux vomica, Pulsatilla, Ruta graveolens, Spigelia, Sulphur

CAFFEINE AND PAIN RELIEVERS

The following over-the-counter and prescription medicines contain caffeine.

Over-The-Counter Medicines
Anacin Tablets and Caplets
Anacin, Maximum Strength Tablets
Arthritis Strength BC Powder
Bayer Select Headache Pain Relief
BC Powder
Excedrin, Aspirin-Free Analgesic Tablets
Excedrin Extra-Strength Analgesic Tablets and Caplets
Midol, Maximum Strength Multi-Symptom Menstrual
   Formula
P-A-C Analgesic Tablets
Vanquish Analgesic Tablets and Caplets

Prescription Medicines
B-A-C
Damason-P
Darvon Compound and Darvon Compound-65
Esgic
Fioricet and Fioricet with codeine
Fiorinal and Fiorinal with codeine 3
Synalgos-DC

Analgesic-dependent Headaches

Headaches from analgesic abuse are similar to those of mixed headaches in that they combine symptoms of migraine and tension headaches. The dependence on analgesics usually arises from an insidious cycle of headache pain, anxiety about pain, and increasing doses of pain medication that spirals out of control. In other words, the more you take, the less it helps; the less it helps, the more anxious you become; the more anxious you become, the greater the likelihood of a headache. And if the medications you use contain caffeine, the problem is compounded by the ill effects of caffeine dependence.

If you get headaches on a daily basis and are taking the maximum dosage of over-the-counter medications to relieve them, or have moved on to more and stronger prescription medications to prevent headache, you are caught in this cycle. Review your headache and medication patterns carefully with your doctor as well as your homeopath. You should make every effort to wean yourself off the medications, and be carefully monitored while you do it. Once your system is clear of the drugs, you can treat any headaches that arise on an as-needed basis.

If you suffer with analgesic-dependent headaches, your diary entries will include some or all of these symptoms:

Onset: Daily. From anxiety or fear.

Location: Temples and sides. May be localized.

Sensation: Dull, diffuse aching.

Concomitants: Nausea, trembling, pallor, tinnitus (ringing or buzzing in the ears).

Mentals and Generals: Depression, anxiety disorders, sleep disturbances.

Homeopathic remedies that may be helpful for analgesic-dependent headaches include:

Aconitum napellus, Argentum nitricum, Calcarea carbonica, China officinalis, Gelsemium, Ignatia, Iris versicolor, Kali bichromicum, Magnesia phosphorica, Natrum muriaticum, Nux vomica, Pulsatilla, Sulphur

Pathological Headaches

Headaches can be triggered by physiological changes such as fluctuations in brain chemicals or hormonal levels, or by illnesses, such as hypertension or inflammatory disease. Although the changes may be normal—as with the hormonal changes that occur throughout a woman's menstrual cycle, or with a flood of adrenaline in response to being startled—the pain of headache is not normal and is therefore classified as a pathology, an illness.

If you have an underlying illness such as arthritis, it is important to keep your doctor informed of any alternative treatments you intend to use and of any results you experience. You may get the best results from a combination of treatments, and it is unwise to abandon any useful practice when investigating another.

Premenstrual Headaches

About two-thirds of the women who seek treatment for headaches report that their pain is related to their menstrual cycles, and some 14 percent of them get migraines. The headache usually occurs in the premenstrual portion of their cycles, and, even if it is not an actual migraine, the pain can be as intense as a migraine and may be accompanied by migraine symptoms, such as nausea or lassitude.

The pain seems to be due to fluctuations of estrogen. In high estrogen states, such as pregnancy, headache is virtually absent. The rapid fall in estrogen during the premenstrual period is thought to be the headache trigger.

If you suffer with premenstrual headaches, your diary entries will include some or all of these symptoms:

Onset: Periodic, every month just prior to menses or at ovulation.

Location: Front of head, temples, or generalized.

Sensation: Throbbing, pounding, head feels full and heavy.

Concomitants: Migraine symptoms: nausea, visual disturbances, pallor, trembling. Gastrointestinal disturbances: constipation, diarrhea, stomach cramps.

Modalities

> *Worse*: Motion, light. Smell of food may provoke vomiting or aggravate nausea.
>
> *Better*: At onset of menses or during period. Warmth. Pressure.
>
> *Mentals and Generals*: Irritable, short-tempered. Tearful, sentimental. Poor concentration. Listless or restless.

Homeopathic remedies that may be helpful for premenstrual headaches include:

Argentum nitricum, Bryonia, Colocynthis, Lachesis, Magnesia phosphorica, Pulsatilla

Melilotus (sweet clover), a remedy not detailed in the Materia Medica in this book because of its limited use in other kinds of headache, may be particularly helpful for premenstrual headache. If you get migraines or throbbing, pounding, migraine-like "sick" headaches in the premenstrual portion of your cycle and the pain stops or eases when the flow starts, try Melilotus.

Other symptoms for this remedy are retching, vomiting, pallor, cold extremities (hands and feet), visual disturbances (black spots before your eyes), an undulating sensation in your brain, constipation, feeling smothered (breathless) from slight exertion, and sore joints (especially the knees).

Hypertension (High Blood Pressure) Headaches

If you have hypertension, it is more critical that your blood pressure be managed appropriately than that you avoid headache. Unfortunately, some blood pressure medicines trigger headache and some headache medicines aggravate high blood pressure; so, it is especially important that you not rely on self-treatment but rather work with a qualified and sympathetic doctor to find the best balance of treatments for optimum health. Talk to your doctor before trying any homeopathic remedies and keep her informed about the effects you experience.

Diligent practice of dietary changes (reducing salt intake), consistent (if mild) exercise, and stress management can help reduce the amount of medication needed to manage your blood pressure.

If you suffer with hypertension headaches, your diary entries will include some or all of these symptoms:

Onset: Headache starts in the morning or you awaken with the pain. After stress. After certain foods (*see*: The Migraine Diet).

Location: Back of the head or generalized.

Sensation: Dull ache. Pain feels like a "hat band" around the head.

Modalities

Worse: In the morning.

Concomitants: Nausea and vomiting.

Homeopathic remedies that may be helpful for hypertension headaches include:

Aconitum napellus, Apis mellifica, Belladonna, Colocynthis, Gelsemium, Lachesis, Sanguinaria

Inflammatory Disease

Inflammation, literally "to flame within," is defined by four factors: redness, heat, swelling, and pain. It is a defensive reaction in which your blood vessels dilate, resulting in swelling—intended to isolate the injury or pathogens (germs)—and pain—to remind you to hold still and not injure yourself any further. The redness and heat come from increased circulation as your blood cells work to repair the damage or kill the intruders. (Body heat comes from the friction of your blood cells against the vessel walls.)

This defensive activity can feel like an illness in and of itself, and particular kinds of inflammation define certain diseases. Illnesses that end in "itis"—arthritis, sinusitis, appendicitis, hepatitis—are inflammatory diseases. Headache, loss of appetite, and generalized discomfort are typical concomitants of inflammation.

Arthritis/Cervical Spondylitis

Inflammation of the joints and muscles in your head and neck due to cervical spondylitis, a form of arthritis, can cause a headache with symptoms similar to those of tension headaches. In cervical spondylitis, bony deposits form on the neck portion of the spine. These deposits inhibit motion and can impinge on the nerves, which can be very painful. In reaction, you will try to hold your head and neck still and that muscle tension compounds the original problem. In some cases, the muscle tension may be severe enough to be mistaken for arthritis, and tests to confirm the illness are advised. Often in arthritis the pain is worse with movement but the illness is better with consistent moderate exercise.

If you suffer with arthritis headaches, your diary entries will include some or all of these symptoms:

Location: Back of the head.

Sensation: Dull ache. Shooting pain.

Concomitants: Stiff neck and shoulders.

Modalities

　　Worse: With movement. Damp and/or cold weather.

Homeopathic remedies that may be helpful for arthritis headaches include:

Arsenicum album, Bryonia, Calcarea carbonica, Ferrum phosphorica, Gelsemium, Magnesia phosphorica, Natrum muriaticum, Nux vomica, Spigelia

Rhus toxicodendron (poison ivy), a remedy not detailed in the Materia Medica in this book because of its limited use in other kinds of headache, may be helpful for arthritis headache. The defining characteristics for this remedy are *stiffness* and *better with motion.*

Rhus tox is sometimes called the "rusty hinge" remedy. It is helpful in conditions where stiffness contributes to pain, and the pain and stiffness are progressively relieved by movement. Typically the stiffness is worse in the morning, occurs in the neck or lower back, and provokes restlessness in the search for relief. A Rhus tox headache centers in the base of the skull or starts in the forehead, then creeps back and settles in the base of the skull.

Cold or Flu Headaches

The head congestion that typically accompanies colds, flus, and sinus infections (see below) can also trigger headache. When repertorizing these headaches, pay particular attention to the concomitant symptoms and the mentals and generals. These will be the best guides to identifying an appropriate remedy. The Mentals and Generals that people manifest during a cold or the flu are so varied, idiosyncratic, and contradictory that to try to summarize them here would be more confusing than helpful. Refer to the listings in the Materia Medica (Part Three) for specific information on the recommended remedies.

If taken at the first glimmer of a cold, Aconitum napellus may abort it. Similarly, oscillococcinum, a remedy not detailed in this book because of its limited use in headache treatment, may prevent flu. (Homeopathic flu prevention remedies may be marketed under names like

Flu Solution or Flu Stopper.) Once a cold or the flu takes hold, however, you'll be treating the symptoms as they arise.

If you suffer with headaches from a cold or the flu, you will experience some or all of these symptoms:

Onset: Sudden or gradual, with infection.

Location: Front of head or generalized.

Sensation: Throbbing, pounding. Head feels hot, full, heavy.

Concomitants: Chills or fever. Sweating. Body aches, stiff joints. May be restless or so sleepy you cannot stay awake. Respiratory complaints: coughs, difficulty breathing, sore throat. Skin may be flushed or pale. Eyes painful, bloodshot, tearing.

Homeopathic remedies that may be helpful for headaches from a cold or the flu include:

Aconitum napellus, Argentum nitricum, Arnica, Arsencium album, Belladonna, Bryonia, China officinalis, Colocynthis, Ferrum phosphoricum, Gelsemium, Ignatia, Kali bichromicum, Lachesis, Lycopodium, Magnesia phosphorica, Nux vomica, Spigelia, Sulphur

Sinusitis

Headache is a primary symptom of inflamed or infected sinuses. The pain centers in the face behind the eyes, forehead, nose, and cheekbones. It can be incapacitating and will last as long as the underlying condition does.

Chronic sinus trouble can result from poor drainage due to structural problems in the nose and sinuses. When an allergy or infection triggers mucus production, the sinuses clog and fester. In advanced cases, surgery to correct the bone structure may be advised.

If you suffer with headaches from sinusitis, your diary entries will include some or all of these symptoms:

Onset: From infection, such as a cold, or allergy.

Location: Facial mask: eyes, forehead, nose, cheekbones.

Sensation: Constant deep dull ache.

Concomitants: Thick, greenish or yellow nasal discharge. Postnasal drip. Coughing. Nausea.

Modalities

Better: Hot compresses. Humidifying the sinuses.

Homeopathic remedies that may be helpful for headaches from sinusitis include:

Aconitum napellus, Apis mellifica, Belladonna, Bryonia, Calcarea carbonica, Colocynthis, Ignatia, Kali bichromicum, Lachesis, Lycopodium, Magnesia phosphorica, Natrum muriaticum, Pulsatilla

Trauma

Caution: Any headache that follows an injury to the head, neck, or back *must* be evaluated by a physician. Undiagnosed internal damage may be crippling or fatal.

Headaches from head or neck injuries may trigger headaches in someone who was previously headache-free or aggravate headaches in someone who already suffers from them. The headaches may begin within hours of the accident or take several weeks to manifest. They may persist for months or years and can mimic migraine or chronic tension headaches.

Trauma headaches typically resist treatment and the tendency to abuse analgesics in the search for relief should be guarded against.

If you suffer with headaches after an injury, you may experience some or all of these symptoms:

Onset: After an injury, especially whiplash or a blow to the head. Daily or episodic.

Location: Back of the head.

Sensation: Migraine-like, throbbing, pounding, pulsating, or similar to tension headache, a constant dull ache.

Concomitants: Neck pain. Dizziness. Fatigue. Tinnitus (ringing or buzzing in the ears). Hypersensitive to noise or light.

Modalities

Better: Hot applications.

Mentals and Generals: Unable to concentrate. Impaired comprehension of new or complex material. Anxious, irritable, short-tempered. Easily frustrated. Insomnia. Depression.

Homeopathic remedies that may be helpful for headaches from trauma include:

Aconitum napellus, Apis mellifica, Arnica, Bryonia, China officinalis, Ferrum phosphoricum, Gelsemium, Iris versicolor, Lachesis, Magnesia phosphorica, Natrum muriaticum, Nux vomica, Spigelia, Sulphur

ENVIRONMENTAL HEADACHES

Airborne allergens (such as dust or pollen), bright lights, loud noises, strong odors, even changes in the weather can provoke headaches in sensitive people. As with hangover headaches, the best treatment is prevention—avoid the headache trigger altogether. This approach may not be possible, but you should take whatever steps are necessary to limit your exposure to factors that injure your health.

ENVIRONMENTAL TOXINS
THAT MAY TRIGGER HEADACHE

Carbon monoxide (tobacco smoke, car exhaust, fumes
  from a leaky furnace)
Coal fumes
Dust (house dust, metal dust, grain and wood dust)
Dyes
Factory smoke
Fluorocarbons
Glues (industrial glues used in carpets, laminates,
  flooring)
Insecticides, pesticides, and weed killers
Motor oil
Paints and solvents
Perfumes and deodorizers
Pollen
Polyvinylchloride

Airborne Allergens and Headaches

Trees, grasses, weeds, and flowers release their pollen at
particular times of the year. If you get headaches at specific times of the year and also experience allergy symptoms such as itchy watery eyes, wheezing and sneezing,
or congestion, you probably have a seasonal allergy.

If, however, your symptoms are site-specific, that is,
you experience them after you have been in a particular
place, regardless of the time of year, you likely have a
perennial allergy. Common allergens that provoke perennial allergies are dust, dust mites, pet dander, and environmental toxins, such as formaldehyde or Formalin (which
you may encounter in an office more than at home).

There is some controversy about the connection
between allergies and headache. Careful analysis of the
entries in your headache diary will help you identify
whether allergies are a factor in your headache pattern.

If you suffer with headaches associated with airborne allergens, your diary entries will include some or all of these symptoms:

Onset: Seasonal.

Location: Facial mask: Forehead, eyes, nose, cheek-bones.

Sensation: Pain can mimic migraine, sinus, or tension headache. Pounding, throbbing, pulsating. Constant dull ache.

Concomitants: Watery eyes. Itchy eyes, nose, ears, mouth, throat. Sneezing. Nasal congestion. Post-nasal drip. Nasal mucus may be clear and watery, or thick and green or yellow.

Homeopathic remedies that may be helpful for headaches associated with airborne allergens include:

Aconitum napellus, Apis mellifica, Belladonna, Calcarea carbonica, Colocynthis, Kali bichromicum, Lycopodium, Pulsatilla, Ruta graveolens, Sanguinaria, Spigelia, Sulphur

Allium cepa (red onion), a remedy not detailed in this book because of its limited use in other headaches, may be especially helpful for headaches associated with airborne allergens. If your primary symptoms include copious, watery nasal discharge; burning, stinging, tearing eyes; sneezing; a cough, hoarseness, or laryngitis; and pain localized in your forehead, try Allium cepa.

Food-related Headaches

Many people find that particular foods play a role in their headache patterns. Determining whether you are allergic in the medical sense of the word is a job for an allergist, but you can track and identify foods or eating patterns that provoke your headaches with the headache diary (*see*: The Migraine Diet and Using the Headache Diary), then test whether eliminating them from your diet stops the headaches.

Some people are sensitive to the food's temperature, rather than to the food itself. Very cold foods or drinks provoke headache more commonly than hot foods and drinks. After identifying a food or food category that is troublesome, it may be useful to test whether the serving temperature is a factor.

Food Allergies and Headaches

Allergies and sensitivities are physiological reactions in which your immune system reacts to a normally benign substance such as a strawberry as though it were a pathogen, a substance capable of producing a disease. The distinction between an allergy and a sensitivity is mostly a matter of the severity with which your immune system reacts. On the high end of the scale is an allergic reaction called *anaphylaxis* or *anaphylactic shock*. This is an allergic reaction severe enough to be fatal unless immediate medical intervention is obtained. Sensitivities, including food sensitivities, are at the lower end of the scale. If you breathe, touch, or eat something that disagrees with you, it's not a fight to the death. You are more likely to feel "out of sorts"—headachy, mildly stuffed up, or a little queasy—for a relatively short period of time. Allergies tend to run in families and some headaches—migraine for example—also have a genetic component. If both illnesses occur in your family, it increases the likelihood of a connection between an allergen and your headache.

Over the years of research into headache, a list of foods that are implicated as triggers has been compiled (*see*: The Migraine Diet). Many of these are processed foods that can complicate other illnesses as well, but some are not. If any of the known food triggers are present in your diet, record your reactions in your diary. Be aware that while you may not be sensitive to one specific food, you may be sensitive to another in that food category. Also, some people are sensitive to the food's temperature, rather than to the food itself. Ice cream or other ice-cold foods and drinks are a common trigger. Before deciding you are allergic to dairy foods, review whether it's the temperature, rather than the lactose, that is giving you trouble. Once you have identified foods that trigger headaches, removing them from your diet should remove headaches from your life.

If you suffer with food-related headaches, your diary entries will include some or all of these symptoms:

Onset: After eating or drinking.

Location: Localized or generalized.

Sensation: Migraine or migraine-like pain. Dull ache.

Concomitants: Nausea, bloating, gas. Itchy mouth, throat, eyes, or skin.

Homeopathic remedies that may be helpful for food-related headaches include:

Aconitum napellus, Argentum nitricum, Calcarea carbonica, Ignatia, Lycopodium, Pulsatilla, Sanguinaria, Spigelia, Sulphur

Cold foods or drinks: Arsenicum album, Calcarea carbonica, Lycopodium, Pulsatilla, Spigelia, Sulphur

Dairy products: Apis mellifica (if you crave milk), Calcarea carbonica

Fruit: Ignatia

Fruit, citrus: Arsenicum album

Red wine: Sanguinaria

Fasting and Indigestion Headaches

Skipping meals can cause a form of rebound headache. Similarly, indigestion from overeating or eating disagreeable foods may be accompanied by headache. Amending unwholesome eating habits will improve your overall health as well as aiding in headache prevention.

If you suffer with food-related headaches, your diary entries will include some or all of these symptoms:
Onset: After eating or drinking.
Location: Localized or generalized.
Sensation: Migraine or migraine-like pain. Dull ache.
Concomitants: Nausea, bloating, gas. Itchy mouth, throat, eyes, or skin.

Homeopathic remedies that may be helpful for headaches from fasting include:
Calcarea carbonica, China officinalis, Colocynthis, Lachesis, Lycopodium, Sulphur.

Homeopathic remedies that may be helpful for headaches that accompany indigestion include:
Aconitum napellus, Argentum nitricum, Arsenicum album, Colocynthis, Iris versicolor, Lycopodium, Magnesia phosphorica, Nux vomica

Weather-related Headaches
Some people, especially those who are prone to migraines, will get headaches when the weather changes or when the seasons change. Any change can cause pain, but heat and/or humidity are generally more troublesome than cold, dry conditions, as are changes from cool seasons to warm seasons or from dry to rainy. Pressure shifts from low to high can also trigger headache in sensitive people. Rapid, alternating shifts of temperature and humidity, as when going in and out of air-conditioned buildings in the summer, can also spark a headache.

If you suffer with weather-related headaches, your diary entries will include some or all of these symptoms:

Onset: Change of temperature or humidity. Change of season.

Location: Front of head or generalized.

Sensation: Pounding, throbbing, bursting, pulsating. Constant dull ache.

Modalities

Better: In stable environment.

Homeopathic remedies that may be helpful for weather-related headaches include:

Change of season: Colocynthis, Lachesis

Cold: Calcarea carbonica, Gelsemium

Dampness: Arsenicum album, Calcarea carbonica

Heat and sun: Belladonna, Ferrum phosphoricum, Lachesis, Sanguinaria, Spigelia

Using the Headache Diary

Why Use a Diary?

The goal of the diary is to discover how and why the pain starts. The more information you can give to a practitioner, the more accurately you can be treated. Transcribe the questions on the pages that follow into a notebook or photocopy enough of them to track your headaches for at least one month. People who get headaches less frequently may need to maintain the diary for several months.

Headaches have emotional as well as physical triggers. Be frank about what is going on with you. Knowing that you get headaches after an emotional upset—whether it's anger, anxiety, fear, frustration, or embarrassment—or from overeating, poor nutrition, smoking, or drug use is significant in treating them.

Describe your headaches vividly, draw pictures, wax poetic. It makes a difference if the pain is bursting or crushing, prickly or dull, spasmodic or constant. Concomitant symptoms—if you feel hot (with or without a measurable fever) or chilled, if the pain is in the front of your head or the back—influence remedy choices.

How you cope with the pain is also significant. The coping patterns of migraine and cluster sufferers, for example, are poles apart. Migraineurs generally take to their beds and stay as still and quiet as possible until the pain stops. The pain of a cluster headache, however, typically causes a sufferer to cry out and drives him into desperate activity—pacing the floor or head banging—in the search for relief. Your pattern probably falls somewhere between them. Make notes about how you felt before the headache started and after it ended.

Undoubtedly, you are not going to want to do this while you are in pain. Make the notes as soon as you can after the headache subsides. If you let too much time elapse, you'll forget some things that could be important.

Finally, since wellness is the goal, it is helpful to give the homeopath some idea of how you are when you are well. As described in Part One, a homeopath will ask a wide range of questions about your life and general well-being. If you are innately self-directed and energetic, you will benefit from different remedies than someone whose nature is yielding and placid—even if your physical symptoms are identical.

ANALYZING YOUR HEADACHE PATTERNS

When you have records for about half a dozen headaches, read through your notes and look for patterns. Use a highlighting marker to identify situations that repeat or have escalated.

Do the headaches occur at particular times of the day, week, or month? Is the pain worse in the morning or at night? Are they associated with any foods or beverages? Did they begin after an argument with your spouse or a hard day at work? What made the workday so difficult? What was the fight about? Did you take any medication for the pain? Did it help? Have you started taking three or four aspirin at a time to get the same relief you used to have with one or two? Are the headaches more frequent or do they last longer?

Review the patterns with your doctor and homeopath. In addition to finding an appropriate remedy, consider changing your habits to circumvent headaches. Dietary changes, stress management, and consistent mild exercise will improve your overall health and may help to reduce the frequency and intensity of your headaches.

In addition to the kinds of questions described in Part One, a homeopath (or your doctor) may ask some or all of the following:

Onset, Frequency, and Duration
Do you know what triggered the headache?
  An injury? Dental work? Stress? Missed meals?
Have you had a headache like this before?
Does exertion (lifting, running, straining, sex) affect your
  headache?
Is your headache associated with your menstrual cycle?
Are any foods associated with your headache?
Does drinking alcohol cause or aggravate your headache?
Does not drinking coffee or soda cause or aggravate your
  headache?

Location and Sensation
Where is the pain?
  Left side? Right? Front? Back? A band around the
  head? In one spot as though a nail were driven into
  your skull?
Describe the pain.
  Is it sharp or dull? Throbbing or a constant ache?
  Burning? Shooting? Pushing outward or pressing
  inward?
Do you have any changes in vision before or during your
headache?

Blurred vision? Hypersensitivity to light? Floating spots? Flashing lights?

Modalities

At what time of day or night do you feel worse (or better)?

What relieves your symptoms and/or makes you feel better?

What aggravates your symptoms and/or makes you feel worse?

Concomitants

Is there any change in your body temperature (with or without a measurable fever)?

Is there a change in your physical appearance?

Flushed? Pale? Bluish or purplish patches?

Are your neck, shoulder, or arm muscles sore during the headache?

Is the eye on the painful side teary and inflamed?

Do you have ear or hearing problems, such as tinnitus (ringing or buzzing in the ears), drainage, or stuffiness in either ear?

Do you have any facial pain, an achy jaw, or congestion along with your headache?

Have you noticed any paralysis, muscle weakness, numbness, swallowing problems, or speech changes during your headache?

Any digestive complaints?

Indigestion? Nausea? Vomiting? Constipation or diarrhea?

Belching or flatulence?

Mentals and Generals

Has your mood changed?

Irritable? Anxious or fearful? Giddy? Talkative? Sad?

Is there a change in your energy level?

Listless? Restless? Easily fatigued?

Is your appetite or thirst affected?
Are you sleeping well?

Treatment History
Has it been over 18 months since you visited a dentist?
Have you had medical tests for headaches (X ray, CAT scan, MRI)?
Has your headache pattern changed in the last six months?
Do you take medication several times a week for your headache?
Do you get a severe headache if you stop your headache medication?

DIARY SUMMARY

If you get several headaches in a week, do weekly summaries for a month. If your headaches are less frequent, summarize when you have information from four to six episodes. Note the age you were when your headaches first started and whether you have any close relatives who get headaches as well as what kind of headaches they get.

Headache Analysis
Total number of headaches   in one month:
in one week:
     Number of days between headaches:
Number of morning headaches: afternoon headaches:
Number of all-day headaches:
Number of multi-day headaches:
Number of days duration:
Number of headaches affecting the whole head:
. . . affecting one side or a portion of the head:
How many of these headaches were debilitating?
How many were mild to moderately intense?
Did any of the headaches wake you at night?

. . . wake you in the morning?
. . . keep you from falling asleep at night?
Average duration of headache (minutes, hours, days):
Average intensity of pain:
                          (mild) 1 2 3 4 5 6 7 8 9 (severe)

Headache Diary Form

Date: _____

Warning signs: _____

Onset: _____

Time begun: _____

Time ended: _____

Location: _____

Sensation/Type of pain: _____

Intensity of pain:
(mild) 1 2 3 4 5 6 7 8 9 (severe) _____

Effect of treatment: _____

Better with: _____

Worse with: _____

Concomitants: _____

Mentals & Generals: _____

Treatment or medication taken: _____

Comments/Triggers: _____

Headache Diary Form

Date: _____

Warning signs: _____

Onset: _____

Time begun: _____

Time ended: _____

Location: _____

Sensation/Type of pain: _____

Intensity of pain:
(mild) 1 2 3 4 5 6 7 8 9 (severe) _____

Effect of treatment: _____

Better with: _____

Worse with: _____

Concomitants: _____

Mentals & Generals: _____

Treatment or medication taken: _____

Comments/Triggers: _____

PART THREE

THE MATERIA MEDICA, A CATALOG OF REMEDIES

HOW TO USE THIS SECTION

The following section is the *Materia Medica* (Latin for "Materials of Medicine"). It is a catalog of 25 remedies demonstrated to be helpful for various kinds of headache. In this book the Medica is divided into two sections; the information in each section is essentially the same, but it is organized differently. The classic homeopathic references describe the remedies in narrative lists arranged by category (location, sensation, modalities, etc.), and you'll find that here as well. However, when trying to decide between two remedies, it can be helpful to be able to compare the descriptions side-by-side, and so the information is also given in chart form.

Each remedy description follows the same format. At the top of the page is the full name of the remedy, its common name, and its standard abbreviation. Below the remedy name is a list of symptoms divided into specific categories that help in deciding which to choose for a particular condition. The categories are:

Helpful for: A list of the kinds of headaches for which the remedy can be used.

Onset: A description of how the symptoms begin, for example: Slow or fast? From a stimulus such as food or weather? From emotional shock or physical exertion?

Location: Where the pain localizes or how it moves, for example: "starts in base of skull spreads to forehead" or "behind jaw hinges."

Sensation: The specific ways you feel the pain. Typical descriptions include: bursting, crushing, dull, knifelike, as if pierced by a nail. Note also the severity of the pain. Is it incapacitating or tolerable? Mild or excruciating?

Modalities: What makes you or your symptoms feel better? What makes you or your symptoms feel worse?

Concomitants: These are symptoms that you may experience in addition to the headache, for example: nausea, vomiting, muscle pain, real or perceived changes in body temperature (fever/chills).

Mentals & Generals: These are symptoms such as forgetfulness or confusion, changes in your emotional state (irritable, whiny, desires solitude, desires company), and alterations in your sleep patterns or appetite (food cravings or aversions).

A short summary follows the list. The summary highlights the characteristic symptoms of a particular remedy, the kind of personality structure that usually matches the remedy, and information to help you decide between remedies with similar profiles. Homeopathy often uses metaphor and descriptive comparisons—pain is described as "like a thousand little hammers" or "like lightning;" pain may cause a patient to "den up like a bear" or symptoms may erupt "volcanically." These descriptions form an accurate and recognizable profile of illness and help to define appropriate remedies.

Choosing a Remedy

You know how it hurts when you get a headache. You know whether the pain localizes on one side of your head or if it settles in the base of your skull. You know if it was triggered by eating a particular food or by skipping a meal, by rainy weather or too much sun. You know if it's your weekend headache or your every-three-days headache. If you suffer from chronic headaches, you will know from the first hint of a symptom whether this one will be protracted and incapacitating or transient and tolerable. If you get headaches you know these things— and this knowledge will help you determine an appropriate homeopathic remedy.

Review your headache diary and your responses to the diagnostic interview, organizing your symptoms in the same categories that are given in the Materia Medica. When you consider a remedy, you are looking for a description that matches the greatest number of your particular symptoms. It is unlikely that you will experience the full range of symptoms described, so don't discount a remedy that includes symptoms you are not experiencing. For example, you may get headaches when you are under stress trying to make a deadline. You list your symptoms like this:

Onset: From deadline stress.
Location: Temples. Sometimes radiates across forehead. Eyestrain. Stiff neck.
Sensation: Long slow waves of pain. Prickly pain.
Concomitants: Blurred vision (eyestrain). Nausea.
Better: Cold drinks. Keeping the window open or sitting in front of a fan.
Worse: At night.

Looking through the Materia Medica you will find that Argentum nitricum (Arg-n) and Iris versicolor (Iris) encompass symptoms of stress, blurred vision (eyestrain), nausea, and worse at night. Both are better with cold: Arg-n with "Cold. Fresh air" (the open window and fan), Iris with "Cold drinks." Both include vomiting, which despite the nausea is not one of your symptoms. Arg-n includes trembling and a craving for sweets, which you are not experiencing. You also don't have nerve pains throughout your face and intense ringing or buzzing in your ears, which are Iris symptoms. Neither description includes stiff neck. Nevertheless, these two remedies are strong candidates, and the deciding factors will be more specific regarding location, sensation, and onset.

Location: Arg-n tends to be right-sided or frontal pain, and Iris is more commonly left-sided. Your forehead and temples (left and right side) hurt. Arg-n includes both (right side, front). Iris includes one (left side).

Sensation: Arg-n pain increases and decreases gradually (matching your "long slow waves of pain"). The "prickly" quality of the pain is a symptom that could go either way. It suggests the nerve pain of Iris, but since it is localized in your forehead and not "over the face," it could be considered part of the Arg-n picture.

Onset: Thinking about the onset, you realize that your headaches come on while you are working, which is another characteristic of Arg-n. Iris headaches arise when the stress ends.

For a headache with this particular constellation of symptoms, Arg-n is a better overall match than Iris.

SUMMARY OF REMEDIES FOR HEADACHE TYPES

Airborne Allergens Headaches

Aconitum napellus, Apis mellifica, Belladonna, Calcarea carbonica, Colocynthis, Kali bichromicum, Lycopodium, Pulsatilla, Ruta graveolens, Sanguinaria, Spigelia, Sulphur

Arthritis Headaches

Apis mellifica, Arsenicum album, Bryonia, Calcarea carbonica, Ferrum phosphoricum, Gelsemium, Kali bichromicum, Magnesia phosphorica, Natrum muriaticum, Nux vomica, Spigelia

Cluster Headaches

Aconitum napellus, Argentum nitricum, Belladonna, Bryonia, China officinalis, Ignatia, Lachesis, Nux vomica, Ruta graveolens, Sanguinaria, Spigelia

Cold or Flu Headaches

Aconitum napellus, Argentum nitricum, Arnica, Arsenicum album, Belladonna, Bryonia, China officinalis, Colocynthis, Ferrum phosphoricum, Gelsemium, Ignatia, Kali bichromicum, Lachesis, Lycopodium, Magnesia phosphorica, Nux vomica, Spigelia, Sulphur

Exertion Headaches

Aconitum napellus, Argentum nitricum, Arnica, Arsenicum album, Belladonna, Bryonia, Calcarea carbonica, Iris versicolor, Natrum muriaticum, Nux vomica, Sulphur

Eyestrain Headaches

Argentum nitricum, Arnica, Gelsemium, Natrum muriaticum, Ruta graveolens

Food-related Headaches

Aconitum napellus, Apis Mellifica, Argentum nitricum, Arsenicum album, Calcarea carbonica, China officinalis, Colocynthis, Ignatia, Iris versicolor, Lachesis, Lycopodium, Magnesia phosphorica, Nux vomica, Pulsatilla, Sanguinaria, Spigelia, Sulphur

Hangover Headaches

Arsenicum album, Nux vomica, Ruta graveolens

Hypertension (High Blood Pressure) Headaches

Aconitum napellus, Apis mellifica, Belladonna, Colocynthis, Gelsemium, Lachesis, Sanguinaria

Migraine Headaches

Argentum nitricum, Arnica, Arsenicum album, Belladonna, Bryonia, Calcarea carbonica, China officinalis, Colocynthis, Gelsemium, Ignatia, Iris versicolor, Kali bichromicum, Lachesis, Natrum muriaticum, Nux vomica, Pulsatilla, Sanguinaria, Spigelia, Sulphur

Mixed Headaches

Aconitum napellus, Apis mellifica, Argentum nitricum, Belladonna, Bryonia, Calcarea carbonica, Colocynthis, Gelsemium, Ignatia, Iris versicolor, Kali bichromicum, Lachesis, Natrum muriaticum, Nux vomica, Pulsatilla, Sanguinaria, Spigelia, Sulphur

Premenstrual Headaches

Apis mellifica, Argentum nitricum, Bryonia, Colocynthis, Lachesis, Magnesia phosphorica, Pulsatilla, Sanguinaria

Rebound Headaches/Analgesics

Aconitum napellus, Argentum nitricum, Calcarea carbonica, China officinalis, Gelsemium, Ignatia, Iris versicolor, Kali bichromicum, Magnesia phosphorica, Natrum muriaticum, Nux vomica, Pulsatilla, Sulphur

Rebound Headaches/Caffeine

Bryonia, Gelsemium, Ignatia, Iris versicolor, Lachesis, Natrum muriaticum, Nux vomica, Pulsatilla, Ruta graveolens, Spigelia, Sulphur

Sinusitis Headaches

Aconitum napellus, Apis mellifica, Belladonna, Bryonia, Calcarea carbonica, Colocynthis, Ferrum phosphoricum, Gelsemium, Ignatia, Kali bichromicum, Lachesis, Lycopodium, Magnesia phosphorica, Natrum muriaticum, Pulsatilla

Tension (Muscle Contraction) Headaches

Aconitum napellus, Apis mellifica, Calcarea carbonica, Colocynthis, Ignatia, Iris versicolor, Lycopodium, Natrum muriaticum, Spigelia

TMJ (Temporomandibular Joint Syndrome) Headaches

Calcarea carbonica, Lachesis, Sanguinaria

Trauma Headaches

Aconitum napellus, Apis mellifica, Arnica, Bryonia, China officinalis, Ferrum phosphoricum, Gelsemium, Iris versicolor, Lachesis, Magnesia phosphorica, Natrum muriaticum, Nux vomica, Spigelia, Sulphur

Weather-related Headaches

Arsenicum album, Belladonna, Calcarea carbonica, Colocynthis, Ferrum phosphoricum, Gelsemium, Lachesis, Sanguinaria, Sulphur

Tension, Vascular, and Mixed Headaches

	Cl	Ex	Eye	Hg	M	Mx	TMJ	T
Aconitum napellus	•	•				•		•
Apis mellifica						•		•
Argentum nitricum	•	•	•		•	•		
Arnica		•	•		•			
Arsenicum album		•		•	•			
Belladonna	•	•			•	•		
Bryonia	•	•			•	•		
Calcarea carbonica		•			•	•	•	•
China officinalis	•				•			
Colocynthis					•	•		•
Ferrum phosphoricum								
Gelsemium			•		•	•		
Ignatia	•				•	•		•
Iris versicolor		•			•	•		•
Kali bichromicum					•	•		
Lachesis	•				•	•	•	
Lycopodium								•
Magnesia phosphorica								
Natrum muriaticum		•	•		•	•		•
Nux vomica	•	•		•	•	•		
Pulsatilla					•	•		
Ruta graveolens	•		•	•				
Sanguinaria	•				•	•	•	
Spigelia	•				•	•		•
Sulphur		•			•	•		

Cl	Cluster	Mx	Mixed
Ex	Exertion	TMJ	Temporomandibular
Eye	Eyestrain		Joint Syndrome
Hg	Hangover	T	Tension
M	Migraine		

Rebound, Pathological, and Environmental Headaches

	Al	Ar	C/F	F-r	Hy	Pm	R/a	R/c	S	Tr	W
Aconitum napellus	•		•	•	•		•		•	•	
Apis mellifica	•	•		•	•	•			•	•	
Argentum nitricum			•	•			•	•			
Arnica			•							•	
Arsenicum album		•	•								•
Belladonna	•		•		•				•		•
Bryonia		•	•			•		•	•	•	
Calcarea carbonica	•	•		•			•		•		•
China officinalis			•	•			•			•	
Colocynthis	•		•	•	•	•			•		•
Ferrum phosphoricum		•	•						•	•	•
Gelsemium		•	•		•		•	•	•	•	•
Ignatia			•	•			•	•	•		
Iris versicolor				•			•	•		•	
Kali bichromicum	•	•	•				•		•		
Lachesis			•	•	•	•		•	•	•	•
Lycopodium	•		•	•					•		
Magnesia phosphorica		•	•	•		•	•		•	•	
Natrum muriaticum		•					•	•	•	•	
Nux vomica		•	•	•			•	•		•	
Pulsatilla	•			•				•	•		
Ruta graveolens	•							•			
Sanguinaria	•			•	•	•					•
Spigelia	•	•	•	•				•		•	
Sulphur	•		•	•			•	•		•	•

Al	Airborne allergens	R/a	Rebound/analgesics
Ar	Arthritis	R/c	Rebound/caffeine
C/F	Cold/Flu	S	Sinusitis
F-r	Food-related	Tr	Trauma
Hy	Hypertension	W	Weather
Pm	Premenstrual		

Materia Medica

ACONITE / ACONITUM NAPELLUS
Acon
(Monkshood)

Helpful for: Airborne allergens, Cluster, Cold/ Flu, Exertion, Food-related, Hypertension, Mixed, Rebound/analgesics, Sinus, Tension, Trauma

Note: Aconite is best used at the first sign of a headache and in its early stages. (If taken soon enough, it may abort the condition entirely.) If relief is incomplete, consider Arsenicum, Belladonna, or Sulphur.

Onset: Sudden, violent, intense, or acute pain. May be precipitated by exposure to a cold draft, or from a shock such as a fright or sudden anger.

Location: Face and head.

Sensation: Pain is intolerable. Heavy, hot, full. Pulsating, bursting. Intracranial pressure, as if the skull were being forced out of the forehead, or as if constricted by a tight band.

Modalities:
Better: In open air, still air. Warmth, perspiring.
Worse: Evening/night. Lying on the affected side. From tobacco smoke. In dry, cold winds. Light touch, light, noise.
Concomitants: Burning sensations. Fever. Dizziness that is worse on rising or shaking the head. Thirst for cold drinks. Upset stomach, Diarrhea or constipation. Weakness.
Mentals & Generals: Great anxiety, fear, and worry that may be out of proportion to the seriousness of the malady. Fear and certainty of imminent death. Restless whether awake or asleep, and tosses around without relief.

The primary characteristic of Aconite is fright and anxiety. An Aconite patient is hypersensitive to sensation, in a hyperalert mental state (unlike Belladonna, which is indicated by delirium and confusion), and consumed by great anxiety, worry, and fear. The fear and anxiety can cause her to exaggerate the severity of the problem—imagining that a headache is caused by a brain tumor, for example—and may be so great that she predicts the time of her death.

APIS MELLIFICA
Apis
(Honeybee)

Helpful for: Airborne allergens, Arthritis/cervical spondylitis, Food-related, Hypertension, Mixed, Premenstrual, Sinus, Tension, Trauma

Note: If relief is incomplete, consider Natrum muriaticum or Lachesis.

Onset: Emotional upset, especially rage, jealousy, disappointment, or fear.

Location: Back of head. Pain that starts on the right side, then moves left.

Sensation: Stinging, burning pain. Sudden stabbing or piercing pains. Back of head feels heavy, dull pain, may extend to neck. Extreme soreness and sensitivity to touch.

Modalities:

Better: Any form of cold—cold wraps, cool or cold drinks, cool bath. Pressure. Open air.

Worse: Any kind of heat—hot applications, hot or warm drinks, a heated room, heat from the sun. Lying down, especially on the painful side, or closing eyes. Motion. In the afternoon, especially between 3 and 5 P.M.

Concomitants: Head bent backwards or bored into pillow. Swelling, or the sensation of swelling. Skin flushed pink (not red). Stiffness. Thirstless, but may crave milk. Dizziness with sneezing.

Mentals & Generals: Drowsy, listless, apathetic, indifferent; but may start, scream, or cry out suddenly. May be whining, tearful, or irritable.

The outstanding characteristics of Apis are puffy swelling, stinging and/or itching, and burning—the symptoms of a bee sting. Crying out from the pain is also a strong indicator. The patient may be restless and dream of flying from place to place. Look for an emotional picture like that of the queen bee—irritable, hypersensitive, jealous, and mean.

ARGENTUM NITRICUM
Arg-n
(Nitrate of Silver)

Helpful for: Cluster, Cold/Flu, Exertion, Eyestrain, Food-related, Migraine, Mixed, Premenstrual, Rebound/analgesics

Onset: Gradual. Emotional upset: fear, anxiety. Extended period of unusual or continued mental exertion, especially if accompanied by anxiety (as for a deadline).

Location: Left or front. Boring pain, left forehead. Frontal region, with enlarged feeling in left eye.

Sensation: Head feels large, as if bones are expanding or separating. Splintery pain. Pain increases and decreases gradually.

Modalities:

Better: Cold. Fresh air. Pressure (head wrapped with a tight band). After belching.

Worse: Intolerant of heat. At night. During menstruation. Left side. Emotional stimulation.

Concomitants: General debility. Coldness and trembling. Blurred vision, eyestrain, sensitive to light. Upper gastric distress, especially if brought on by mental exertion. Nausea, retching and vomiting of bile. Flatulence, explosive belching.

Mentals & Generals: Feels better in fresh air, though headache may be aggravated. Nervous, melancholy, impulsive (wants to do things in a hurry). Has the sense that time is passing slowly. Great desire for sweets or salt, but eating them aggravates the condition and may provoke nausea or vomiting.

Argentum nitricum is particularly well suited to ailments that come on after mental labor or stress, where the stress is accompanied by apprehensiveness and anxiety. Arg-n patients are very mental: they get ideas stuck in their heads and become tormented by them, especially at night. They are generally outgoing, but may suffer "stage fright" in the face of new experiences although they recover quickly.

The desire for sweets or salty foods is more pronounced in Arg-n patients than in Sulphur patients. An Arg-n patient craves strong flavors: very sweet or very salty foods.

ARNICA / ARNICA MONTANA
Arnica, Arn
(Leopard's bane, Mountain daisy)

Helpful for: Cold/Flu, Exertion, Eyestrain, Migraine, Trauma

CAUTION: Head injuries, or headache following an injury, *must* be evaluated by a medical doctor.

Onset: After injury. May also follow an emotional blow—such as grief, remorse, or the sudden realization of financial loss. May follow mental strain or shock. With a cold or the flu.

Location: Generalized.

Sensation: A bruised, sore, achy feeling. Head hot while body feels cold. Head feels contracted.

Modalities:

Better: Lying down or with head low. Open air. Warmth.

Worse: With the least touch or pressure. Motion, physical exertion. Damp cold. Hot sun.

Concomitants: Dizziness, especially when walking. Eyestrain, with bruised sore feeling in eyes. Holds eyes open.

Mentals & Generals: Wants to be left alone, fears being touched. Gloomy. Irritable. May be accident-prone and/or experience a loss of confidence due to accidents.

In most cases of injury give Arnica first to remove the effects of the shock, then follow it with a remedy appropriate to the symptoms. Arnica patients tend to have a high tolerance for pain, sometimes to the point of not realizing how badly they are injured. In any case where the sensation is "achy, bruised, sore all over," give Arnica first.

ARSENICUM ALBUM
Arsenicum, Ars
(Arsenious acid, Arsenic trioxide)

Helpful for: Arthritis/cervical spondylitis, Cold/Flu, Exertion, Food-related, Hangover, Migraine, Weather-related (especially damp or wet weather)

Onset: Exertion, excitement, getting heated. 1–3 P.M. Periodic. Food poisoning.

Location: Forehead and back of head. Right side.

Sensation: Throbbing and burning, waves of pain. Very chilly. Sick, severe headache. Congestion, brain feels loose. Periodic burning pain with restlessness.

Modalities:

Better: Body kept warm and head cool. Head feels better with cold, although cold may aggravate other symptoms. Head elevated. Warmth, warm applications, warm food or drinks. Being kept company.

Worse: Cold food or drink. From eating fruit, especially watery fruits. Physical exertion. Between midnight and 2 A.M. Wet weather. Open air, especially sea air.

Concomitants: Nausea and vomiting, cannot bear the sight or smell of food. Unquenchable thirst, seeks relief with frequent sips. May crave acids, coffee, or milk. Eating or drinking triggers vomiting. Great exhaustion from slight exertion. Head in constant motion, despite aggravation of symptoms. Prostration, pallor. Skin cold.

Mentals & Generals: Great anxiety and restlessness. Seeks relief in motion but is immediately exhausted. Fear, fright, and worry. Fears death and being left alone. Insecure, needy, and fragile. Fears instability, sudden drastic changes. Sensitive to disorder and confusion. Scalp itchy and sensitive, avoids brushing hair.

Outstanding characteristics for Arsenicum are an all-prevailing debility, exhaustion with restlessness, and much worse at night. The patient's history will distinguish Arsenicum from Gelsemium (also used for exhaustion and debility). Arsenicum has a history of great restlessness, feverishness (if not actual fever), and extreme anxiety.

Arsenicum patients are also very self-absorbed; they tend to be clinging, manipulative, possessive, and dependent. While Aconite patients fear death in itself, Arsenicum patients fear the *instability* of it, the not knowing when and how it will occur. Arsenicum people are fastidious about their food and their environments.

BELLADONNA
Bell
(Deadly nightshade)

Helpful for: Airborne allergens, Cluster, Cold/Flu, Exertion, Hypertension, Migraine, Mixed, Sinus, Weather-related (sun, wind or drafts)

Onset: Sudden, severe. Exposure of head to cold (including after a haircut or not wearing a hat). Suppressing flow of nasal mucus.
Location: Predominantly right-sided. Front, right.
Sensation: Throbbing, shooting, stabbing. Hot, burning. Heavy, full. Constricted, as though a band or strap were wrapped around the head. A rush of blood to the painful area.
Modalities:
Better: With warm wraps, bending head backwards, firm pressure applied gradually, semi-erect posture.
Worse: In the light, with cold and drafts, touch, noise, lying down. With motion: jarring, stepping, stooping or bending head forward, rising up. Between 3 P.M. and 9 P.M.
Concomitants: Redness, flushed face. Dilated pupils. Rush of blood to the head. Dizziness when moving head. Blood in nasal mucus. Extremities ice-cold. Congestion. Skin rashes.
Mentals & Generals: Jerking and twitching. Restlessness. Cries out or screams in sleep. Starts awake when falling asleep. Senses hyperacute. Mental excitation. Furious, strikes out in a rage. Delirium, nightmares, may hallucinate. Disinclined to talk. Changeableness; perversity, with tears.

Belladonna acts on the nervous and vascular systems, and on the skin and glands. Its most outstanding characteristics are: sudden and intense pain; pain that comes and goes abruptly (with anxiety about the return of the pain); hot, red, shiny skin; swelling or a feeling of congestion; throbbing; hypersensitivity to light, noise, smells, touch; and restlessness, especially restless sleep. The patient may have a flushed face; glassy, staring eyes; dilated pupils; and a dry mouth but no thirst. Her limbs may jerk or twitch convulsively. Belladonna is also associated with an excited mental state and with delirium, especially if there is fever. It is also useful for the acute early stages of inflammatory illnesses characterized by high fever and severe pain.

The patient may be kept awake by pain from pulsating blood vessels or the sound of heartbeats reverberating in her head. She may grit her teeth and moan or cry out in her sleep because of nightmares. In extreme cases, the patient may hallucinate. When awake, her attention is focused inward; she may seem dazed and unresponsive or speak nonsensically.

BRYONIA
Bry
(Wild hops)

Helpful for: Arthritis/cervical spondylitis, Cluster, Cold/ Flu, Exertion, Migraine, Mixed, Premenstrual, Rebound/ caffeine, Sinus, Trauma

CAUTION: Head injuries, or headache following an injury, *must* be evaluated by a medical doctor.

Onset: Slow, gradual. From cold, washing in cold water when sweating. May wake with a congested headache.

Location: Base of skull. Right side. Frontal headache, especially if sinuses are involved.

Sensation: Bursting, splitting, as if the skull would split open from within. Fullness and heaviness. Throbbing pain on motion. Stabbing pains over the eyes.

Modalities:

Better: Stillness, especially lying still in a dark room. Firm pressure, especially on painful area. Coolness, open air. Patient should avoid cold, however, as it may trigger a headache.

Worse: Slightest motion or any exertion. From light touch. Heat, especially in a warm and stuffy room. Sitting up. Light. After eating. From coughing. In the morning.

Concomitants: Thirsty and dry. Bitter taste in the mouth. May vomit after eating or drinking, especially after warm drinks. Hot head. Red congested eyes; sore eyeballs. Often nosebleed with headache. Nausea and faintness on rising or lifting head. May be constipated.

Mentals & Generals: Peevish, wants to be left alone. Dull mind, slow, sluggish, passive. May feel homesick, even if at home. Headache precedes or accompanies other illnesses. Must keep perfectly still.

The outstanding characteristic of Bryonia is aggravation with motion; any exertion, even moving the eyes or shifting position when sitting or lying down, will increase the pain. Bryonia is sometimes called the "sleeping bear" remedy. The patient prefers "denning up" (being left alone in a dark place) and will be irritable, snappish, or possibly violent if disturbed. A second characteristic is dryness: dry mouth, possibly with cracked lips, dry nose and/or throat, dry cough (especially at night), with great thirst at long intervals with a desire for large quantities.

CALCAREA CARBONICA
Calc, Calc carb
(Carbonate of lime)

Helpful for: Airborne allergens, Arthritis/cervical spondylitis, Exertion, Food-related (dairy), Migraine, Mixed, Rebound/analgesics, Sinus, Tension, TMJ, Weather-related (cold, wet, change of weather)

Onset: Change of weather. Stress, mental exertion.
Location: Pain radiates through head: from forehead to nose, from temples to the jaw, from base of skull to neck.
Sensation: As if a heavy weight were on top of the head. Scalp itches.
Modalities:
Better: Dry climate and weather. Lying still, lying on painful side.
Worse: Change in weather. Cold in every form. Wet weather. Open air. Mental or physical exertion, worry. Apprehensiveness worse in the evening (may be afraid of the dark).
Concomitants: Increased perspiration, night sweats. Cold hands and feet. Dizziness, nausea. Ravenous hunger and craving for indigestible things (chalk, dirt). Aversion to fats. Craves eggs. Eyes sensitive to light, itchy, tearing. Face pale. Large appetites with slow digestion.
Mentals & Generals: Jaded state, mentally or physically, due to overwork, assuming too much responsibility. Feel they need to do everything themselves, others "won't do it right." Generally passive, but may become obstinate, if asked to do something they don't want to do. Easy relapses, interrupted convalescence. Apprehensive, may be afraid of the dark. Forgetful or slow-witted. Insomnia, nightmares.

People who benefit most from Calcarea have a chilly constitution, the slightest cold "goes right through" them. They may feel cold all the time and have trouble keeping warm. They may become ill after being out in the rain. A second outstanding characteristic is localized or general perspiration—head sweats, for example— which may be profuse and smell sour.

CHINA OFFICINALIS / CINCHONA OFFICINALIS
China
(Peruvian Bark)

Helpful for: Cluster, Cold/Flu, Food-related, Migraine, Rebound/analgesics, Trauma

CAUTION: Head injuries, or headache following an injury, *must* be evaluated by a medical doctor.

Onset: Periodic, every other day.

Location: Back of head, base of skull.

Sensation: As if skull would burst. As if the brain were rocking back and forth, banging against the skull. Great pain. Throbbing, possibly extending to the sides of the throat (carotids). Spasmodic headache, with a bruised feeling. Scalp very sensitive.

Modalities:

Better: Firm pressure. Warm room, warm drinks. Must stand or walk.

Worse: Light touch, combing hair, breezes. Lying or sitting. After eating. At night.

Concomitants: Blue circles around eyes. Visual disturbances: bright dazzling illusions, spots or black spots. Intolerant of light. Ringing in the ears. Flushed face. Hungry without appetite, full after a few bites. Slow digestion. Dizzy when walking. Diarrhea.

Mentals & Generals: Apathetic, indifferent, disobedient. Ill-tempered. Averse to company, disposed to hurt the feelings of others. Ideas crowd the mind, preventing sleep. Wakes up confused, dreams continue while awake. Sudden crying and tossing about.

China is useful for people with chronic conditions, especially an illness that has "gone underground." They suffer with unrefreshing sleep and may have dreams of falling from a great height. Like Calcarea, they are very chilly and can't get warm but may experience recurring fevers (every 7–14 days). They feel better in the autumn, but are generally worse in damp, foggy, windy weather.

COLOCYNTHIS
Coloc
(Bitter cucumber)

Helpful for: Airborne allergens, Cold/Flu, Food-related (hunger, fasting, overeating), Hypertension, Migraine, Mixed, Premenstrual, Sinus, Tension, Weather-related (change of season, wind, damp)

Onset: After vexation. Suppressed emotion, especially anger. Hunger, fasting, or chronic overeating. When seasons change.
Location: Left side. Front.
Sensation: Severe pain. Cramping, constriction, contraction. As if clamped with iron bands. As if stabbed by a spear. Pain may be burning, digging, rending, or tearing. Waves of pain. Shooting, lightning-like pain.
Modalities:
Better: Firm pressure. Lying with knees drawn up to chest. Coffee.
Worse: Resting on back, from stooping, moving eyelids. Cold winds. Damp weather.
Concomitants: Dizziness when turning head to the left. Nausea, vomiting. Sore scalp. Burning tears (from eyes). Bitter taste in mouth. Severe abdominal pain or cramping. Muscles cramped and contracted, joints stiff.
Mentals & Generals: Irritable, short-tempered, angry, indignant. Mortification from offense. May scream from the pain.

Colocynthis is marked by spasms and cramping; patients will bend double and writhe with the pain. They are better with hard pressure and may lean against a chair or the wall or press something hard (like a book) against the painful area. Colocynthis is similar to Magnesia phosphorica but more severe, more left-sided, and better with hard pressure (worse heat).

People who benefit from this remedy are embittered by their pain; they want to be left alone and not bothered. They may have a deep suppressed rage or have experienced years of frustration.

FERRUM PHOSPHORICUM
Ferr-p
(Phosphate of iron)

Helpful for: Arthritis/cervical spondylitis, Cold/Flu, Sinus, Trauma (if Arnica is ineffective), Weather-related (sun)

CAUTION: Head injuries, or headache following an injury, *must* be evaluated by a medical doctor.

Onset: Sudden. After overexposure to the sun. From a head cold or from overexertion.

Location: Right side. Forehead to base of skull, especially right side. Crown, sides.

Sensation: Bruised, pressing, or stitching pain. Pulsating, throbbing. May feel a rush of blood to the head. Sensitive to cold. Head hot and full.

Modalities:

Better: Cold air or applications. Lying down. Pressure. Gentle motion. Having hair touched.

Worse: Wrapping up. Motion, jarring, stepping. Coughing. Light, noise. At night.

Concomitants: Stiff neck. Flushed cheeks, a well-defined, circular redness is characteristic. Nosebleed or bleeding gums. Head hot and full. Feet cold. Dizziness, runny nose, vomiting, or sore scalp. Dark circles under eyes. Eyes may feel as if there is sand under the lids.

Mentals & Generals: Sleep is restless and dreamless. The patient may be lighthearted and talkative, making jokes almost as though she were perfectly well. A fever will sap her energy, however, and the cheerfulness and loquacity will fade as she tires. Has a desire for sour things and a thirst for cold water. Night sweats.

Ferrum phosphoricum is the remedy for low grade or generalized symptoms with inflammation. The sudden

onset of Ferr-p differs from those of Aconite and Belladonna in its severity: Aconite and Belladonna are more
severe, very sudden, very intense; Ferr-p is milder and
less distinct (a fever of 99° or 100°, for example).

GELSEMIUM
Gels
(Yellow jasmine)

Helpful for: Arthritis/cervical spondylitis, Cold/Flu, Eyestrain, Hypertension, Migraine, Mixed, Rebound/analgesics, Rebound/caffeine, Sinus, Trauma, Weather-related (damp, fog, before a storm)

CAUTION: Head injuries, or headache following an injury, *must* be evaluated by a medical doctor.

Onset: Slow, gradual. Early morning, peaks in mid-afternoon. Cold. Emotional upsets: fear, grief, embarrassment.

Location: Back of head, base of skull. May originate in the temple and extend to ear, nose, and chin.

Sensation: Dull, heavy ache originating at the base of the skull, may radiate and settle in forehead or throughout the head. A band of pain. Great heaviness of eyelids and above eyes.

Modalities:

Better: Lying propped up by pillows and quite still. Pressure. Sweating; after urination. With stimulants. Fresh air.

Worse: Damp weather, fog, before a storm (falling barometer). Emotion or excitement (especially bad news). In mid-morning (10 A.M.). Mental effort, heat of sun, tobacco smoke.

Concomitants: Profound exhaustion. Great weakness. Trembling. Nausea. Dizziness, originating at base of skull. Thirstless. Eyes glazed, vision blurred or smoky. Pupils dilated. Muscles of neck and shoulders achy and sore.

Mentals & Generals: The outstanding symptom for Gelsemium is extreme fatigue and sleepiness, the patient simply *cannot* stay awake. If awake, the patient is groggy and lethargic. Very dull-witted, can't rally enough energy to think.

Gelsemium differs from Bryonia in the absolute quality of the exhaustion. Bryonia patients are irritable if disturbed; a Gelsemium patient is too tired to be irritable, too tired to sleep, too tired to eat or drink anything.

Gelsemium is especially helpful for viral infections and for elderly people who are susceptible to infections and who are, or believe that they are, frail.

IGNATIA
Ign
(St. Ignatius bean)

Helpful for: Cluster, Cold/Flu, Food-related, Migraine, Mixed, Rebound/analgesics, Rebound/caffeine, Sinus, Tension

Onset: Emotional distress, especially grief, disappointment, embarrassment or shame (as from being scolded), fear, or anger.

Location: Pain in one spot, as if a nail were driven through the side.

Sensation: Head feels hollow and heavy. Feels as if a nail has been driven into one spot.

Modalities:

Better: While eating. Change of position, especially bending forward. Firm pressure. After urination.

Worse: Strong odors, intolerant of tobacco smoke. Coffee. Stooping. Pressure on the painless side. Morning. Open air, after meals, external warmth.

Concomitants: Vomiting, sensation of a lump in the throat. Chills with fever, thirst during chills, chills relieved by warmth. Skin very sensitive to drafts.

Mentals & Generals: Introspective, sad, brooding, tearful. Rejects company. Not communicative. Disappointed, grieving. All the senses are hyperacute. Insomnia from emotional distress, sleeps lightly with troubling dreams. Contradictory conditions are present and significant for diagnosis: nausea relieved by eating; eating intensifies hunger; may crave indigestible things or acid foods. Simple foods, such as fruit may cause indigestion, while heavier foods are easily tolerated.

The primary factor for this remedy is emotional stress, especially disappointment or grief. Ignatia patients are idealistic, perfectionistic, sensitive, and romantic. (Similar to Sulphur, which is idealistic and intellectual.) Their idealism sets up their grief and disappointments. They are very hard on themselves and others. When disappointed, they try to withhold their response in front of others; then when alone, they will break down into deep uncontrollable sobbing which may alternate with hysterical laughing. Consolation makes the person feel worse. (Similar to Natrum muriaticum, except Nat mur is depression whereas Ignatia is frustration.)

Ignatia patients may have paradoxical symptoms—they crave heat when feverish, exotic foods when suffering indigestion. They have spasms and in extreme cases may develop hysterical symptoms—a paralysis not due to nerve damage, for example.

IRIS VERSICOLOR
Iris, Ir-v
(Blue flag)

Helpful for: Exertion, Food-related, Migraine, Mixed, Rebound/analgesics, Rebound/caffeine, Tension, Trauma

CAUTION: Head injuries, or headache following an injury, *must* be evaluated by a medical doctor.

Onset: After relief of stress, especially mental exertion. Periodic.

Location: Front. Right temple.

Sensation: Sick headaches. Scalp feels constricted. Nerve pains over entire face.

Modalities:

Better: Continued motion. Cold Drinks.

Worse: Rest. In the evening and at night.

Concomitants: Preceded by visual symptoms (cloudy or blurred vision). May have blindness during headache. Burning gastric distress; nausea and vomiting (often in early morning, 2–3 A.M.). Intense ringing or buzzing in the ears that drowns out external sounds.

Mentals & Generals: Low-spirited, cranky, fault-finding. Unable to focus attention on anything. Weakness of memory. Loss of appetite. Accelerated pulse. Chilly through the night.

Iris symptoms are burning or acidic: acid vomiting that burns the throat; watery stools that burn the anus. The mouth may feel greasy and scalded, with profuse secretions, ropy saliva, and a sweet taste. The person may have brief bouts of giddiness or dizziness after coming in from outside.

KALI BICHROMICUM
Kali-bi
(Bichromate of Potash)

Helpful for: Airborne allergens, Arthritis/cervical spondylitis, Cold/Flu, Migraine, Mixed, Rebound/analgesics, Sinus

Onset: Preceded by blurred vision.
Location: Frontal pain, usually over eyebrows, may be over one eye. Sinuses in forehead and cheekbones.
Sensation: Blinding headache. Pains migrate quickly. Vertigo with nausea when rising from sitting.
Modalities:
Better: Heat. Slightly better with pressure.
   Worse: Morning. Hot weather.
Concomitants: Thick, sticky, yellowish green mucus that is stringy, ropy, and difficult to expel. Thick, gagging postnasal drip. Loss of sense of smell. Feels as if digestion has stopped. Dislikes water. Vomiting of bright yellow water. Lower back pain. Laryngitis or hoarseness. Joint pains may alternate with gastric trouble (vomiting, diarrhea) or respiratory problems (coughing, breathlessness). Stopped-up ears or earache.
Mentals & Generals: Extreme aversion to light and noise. General weakness. No fever. Wakes from sleep because of choking. Very low-spirited. Feels worst in the very early morning (2–3 A.M.); may wake up coughing.

Severe, intractable congestion is the primary characteristic of this remedy. Nasal mucus may be green or yellow and malodorous; coughs are brassy and produce a sticky mucus. The headache may literally be blinding, and the patient may have tightly localized pain.

LACHESIS
Lach
(Bushmaster or Surucucu snake venom)

Helpful for: Cluster, Cold/Flu, Food-related, Hypertension, Migraine, Mixed, Premenstrual, Rebound/caffeine, Sinus, TMJ, Trauma, Weather-related (sun)

CAUTION: Head injuries, or headache following an injury, *must* be evaluated by a medical doctor.

Onset: Wakes from pain or pain on waking. From sun, springtime.

Location: Left side. Starts left, then moves right.

Sensation: Waves of pain. Bursting, throbbing, pulsating. Weight and pressure. Pressure and burning on the crown.

Modalities:

Better: With onset of discharges, e.g., nasal mucus or menstrual flow. Open air. Cool and cold temperatures. Few clothes and no blankets. Firm pressure may be comforting.

Worse: Movement, change of position. Entering sleep or on waking (ailment comes on during sleep). Light touch, light, noise. Any heat: sun, warm rooms, application, drinks.

Concomitants: Senses are hyperacute, even the touch of clothes on the skin or the pressure of a blanket may be intolerable. Congested head. Nosebleeds. Face is pale (may be mottled or purplish with fever). Trembling. Dizziness, nausea, and vomiting. Visual disturbances: weak vision, flickering, loss of sight. Tearing pain in jaw.

Mentals & Generals: Sleeps into a headache. Extremely talkative, may not complete one thought or sentence before beginning another. Sad in the morning. Restless and uneasy. Jealous, suspicious, and superstitious. Time sense is deranged.

Lachesis patients are overstimulated but repressed. They seethe with suppressed physical and emotional energy, then implode. (Similar to Sulphur, but Sulphur is overstimulated only on the mental plane.) Their jealousy and suspicions undermine their relationships. They tend to abuse alcohol.

The classic reference works list an inability to tolerate the pressure of clothing as a defining Lachesis symptom.

LYCOPODIUM
Lyc
(Club moss)

Helpful for: Airborne allergens, Cold/Flu, Food-related (hunger or fasting), Sinus, Tension

Onset: Gradual. Taking cold. Hunger or fasting. Congestion.

Location: Right side. Pain starts right, moves left.

Sensation: As if temples were screwed toward each other. Throbbing headache after coughing. Pressing pain on crown of head. Tearing pain at base of skull.

Modalities:

Better: Motion. Warm food and drink. Cool air. With head uncovered.

Worse: Between 4–8 P.M. On waking. Heat or warm rooms, warm applications (except throat and stomach which are relieved by warm drinks). Eating, especially cold food or drink and rich foods. Noise. Lying down.

Concomitants: Shakes head without apparent cause. Facial contortions. Gassy, constipation, or diarrhea. Sour belching. Great hunger easily satisfied or arising soon after a large meal. Craves sweets; warm food and drink. Warm drinks relieve stomach discomfort. Night cough.

Mentals & Generals: Nervous excitement and prostration. Wants to be alone, but wants to know that someone is nearby if needed. Cranky on waking, may wake from hunger. Bullying tendency, with bluff and bravado. Fear of failure, of breaking down under stress.

Lycopodium patients attempt to cover an inner sense of inadequacy by putting up fronts, by pretending to be something they're not. An analogy is made with the Cowardly Lion in *The Wizard of Oz,* who hid an inner timidity beneath a mask of bluff and bluster. Lycopodium people tend to be overdeveloped mentally—they believe it is safer to think than to feel.

MAGNESIA PHOSPHORICA
Mag-p
(Phosphate of Magnesia)

Helpful for: Arthritis/cervical spondylitis, Cold/Flu, Food-related, Migraine, Premenstrual, Rebound/analgesics, Sinus, Trauma

CAUTION: Head injuries, or headache following an injury, *must* be evaluated by a medical doctor.

Onset: Sudden, spasmodic.

Location: Right side. Back of head. Pain over eyes, eyebrows.

Sensation: Shooting, stinging, and darting pain. Feels as if brain were liquid, as if parts were changing places. Eyes hot, vision blurred, colored lights before eyes.

Modalities:

Worse: Right side. Cold. Touch. At night.

Better: Always better with warmth. Bending double. Pressure, rubbing.

Concomitants: Fever with chills, chills run up and down spine, with shivering. Darting pains. General muscular weakness. Severe colicky stomachache, with cramping, bloating, and flatulence.

Mentals & Generals: Worse during mental labor. Tired, exhausted, neurotic. Constant lamenting about the pain. Sleepless due to indigestion. Thirst for cold drinks. Appetite is good, but food may have an "off" taste.

Pain that shifts location rapidly and cramping are the defining characteristics of Magnesia phosphorica. (Similar to Colocynthis but more right-sided, less severe, and better with warmth.) Almost any right-sided condition with cramping, spasmodic pain—toothache, backache, stomachache—will respond to this remedy.

NATRUM MURIATICUM
Nat mur
(Chloride of Sodium, Table Salt)

Helpful for: Arthritis/cervical spondylitis, Exertion, Eye-strain, Migraine, Mixed, Rebound/analgesics, Rebound/caffeine, Sinus, Tension, Trauma

CAUTION: Head injuries, or headache following an injury, *must* be evaluated by a medical doctor.

Onset: Mid-morning (10 A.M.). Grief, humiliation. Eye-strain. Periodical.

Location: Right eye, especially. Back of head, extending down spine.

Sensation: Blinding headache. Pounding, as if a thousand small hammers were knocking on the brain. Bursting. Crushing, pressing as if in a vise.

Modalities:

Better: Sleep, sweating. Open air. Cold bathing. Fasting.

Worse: Moving eyes (as when reading). Between 10–11 A.M. Noise. Consolation. Grief. Heat. Sun.

Concomitants: Tongue feels dry, as if it sticks to the roof of the mouth. Mucous membranes dry. Nausea, vomiting. Stitching pains around eyes. Visual disturbances precede headache: zigzag lines and/or flickering lights. Pallor.

Mentals & Generals: Craves salt and salty foods. Must go to bed and be perfectly quiet. May be weepy, but does not let others see it (worse with consolation). Angry from isolation. Consolation aggravates, wants to be alone to cry. Ill effects of fright, grief, anger, etc. Nervous, discouraged, broken down. Depressed, especially in chronic ailments.

Natrum muriaticum patients are personally aloof but have a social conscience and a desire to help others. The root of this is a desire to protect others from being hurt the way they have been hurt. Nat mur is stoical, depressed, and walled-off, but warm whereas Ignatia is irritable, frustrated, and chilly.

There may be a fear of stinging insects, especially bees, or an allergy to insect bites and a hypersensitivity to light and sunlight, even absent an illness. A Nat mur person might wear sunglasses indoors or at night.

NUX VOMICA
Nux-v
(Poison-nut)

Helpful for: Arthritis/cervical spondylitis, Cluster, Cold/ Flu, Exertion, Food-related, Hangover, Migraine, Mixed, Rebound/analgesics, Rebound/caffeine, Trauma

CAUTION: Head injuries, or headache following an injury, *must* be evaluated by a medical doctor.

Note: Nux is said to act best if given in the evening.

Onset: After overindulgence in food, alcohol, or stimulants. Wakes with headache.

Location: Back of head or over eyes.

Sensation: Piercing, sticking, tearing, burning, stinging. Splitting headache, as if a nail were driven into the crown. Sensation of a great weight on the crown. Frontal headache, with a desire to press head against something.

Modalities:

Better: With rest, in the evening. Wet weather. After a bowel movement.

Worse: Much worse in the morning. Mental exertion. Cold, especially cold dry air. Eating, especially overeating. Stimulants. Anger.

Concomitants: Backache worse lying down, must get up and walk. Pain with nausea and sour vomiting. Easy perspiration; least chill or draft causes headache with stuffy or runny nose. Eyes dry, smarting, twitching. Dizziness, retching, hypersensitivity to light, noise, smells.

Mentals & Generals: Chilly person, better with body warm and head cool (for example: wrapped up in blankets but with head uncovered or with a cool or cold compress). Stomach or liver troubles; with piles. Impatient, irritable, argumentative, oversensitive, touchy. Difficulty sleeping due to overactive mind or sensitivity to slight noises.

Typically, a Nux patient is thin, spare, quick, active, nervous, and irritable. He works with his mind—a student or office worker who has mental strains, cares, and anxieties, and who leads a sedentary life. To compensate he will seek out stimulants, such as coffee, or overindulge in sedatives, such as rich foods and alcohol or, in extreme cases, narcotics. Late hours and fitful sleep are a consequence; a thick head, indigestion, and an irritable temper follow in the morning. He may develop a dependency on cathartics to relieve constipation, antacids to soothe a chronically queasy stomach, and/or analgesics for the headache.

Nux patients are easily chilled and avoid drafts and open air. They are very irritable, fault-finding, and quarrelsome, and do not like to be touched. Their symptoms are always much worse in the morning and are aggravated by mental exertion, tobacco, alcohol, coffee, open air.

PULSATILLA
Puls
(Wind flower)

Helpful for: Airborne allergens, Food-related, Migraine, Mixed, Premenstrual, Rebound/analgesics, Rebound/caffeine, Sinus

Onset: Periodic. Premenstrual. After eating ice cream or rich foods. Overeating, overindulgence. Overwork.

Location: Right side (affected eye may tear). Forehead and sinuses.

Sensation: Wandering, stitching pains through head and face, may extend into the teeth. May be worse on the right side, right eye may tear. Pressure, distention, throbbing. Constricting, congestive.

Modalities:

Better: Consolation. Cold, fresh air. Cold applications. Cold food and drink, though not thirsty. Slow motion in open air. Pressure on painful side. Onset of menses.

Worse: Heat. In the evening and at night. Lying or sitting quiet. Motion of eyes, stooping. Pressure on painless side.

Concomitants: Eyes itch, profuse burning tears or bland yellowish discharge. Thirstless. Sour food causes vomiting.

Mentals & Generals: Weepy, clinging. Moody and changeable. Averse to greasy foods and to warm foods and drinks. Slow digestion, heartburn. Sleeps in the afternoon, may sleep with hands over the head. Great desire for company, sympathy, consolation, reassurance of being loved.

The person's disposition and mental state are the deciding factors for the use of this remedy. Pulsatilla is most effective for people with mild, gentle, yielding natures. People who are sentimental and easily moved to tears, whose moods shift "like the wind." Often they will feel better, whatever their ailment, in the open air, especially if there is a light breeze. They like to rest with their heads propped up and are uncomfortable with only one pillow. They may suffer anxiety or fears at night; primarily, they fear being alone. They are easily discouraged, crave company and sympathy, and enjoy being fussed over.

RUTA GRAVEOLENS
Ruta
(Rue-bitterwort)

Helpful for: Airborne allergens, Cluster, Eyestrain, Hangover, Rebound/caffeine

Onset: After prolonged close work such as sewing or reading small print.

Location: Eyes and eyebrows.

Sensation: Pressure deep in the eyes and over the eyebrows. Eyes feel weary while reading. Aching. Pain as from a nail.

Modalities:

Better: Motion. Heat.

Worse: Lying down, sitting still. Cold, wet weather. From overuse. In the morning.

Concomitants: Eyes are red, hot, tired. Blurry vision. Tearing. Nausea (especially with hangover or from eating cold food), or a nauseated feeling not in the stomach—in the throat, for example. Productive cough (thick, yellow mucus). Short of breath, chest feels tight.

Mentals & Generals: Lassitude, weakness, and despair. Restless from the pain. Feel dissatisfied within themselves.

Ruta works well on tendons, cartilage, and the periosteum (the membrane that covers bones). It is distinct from Arnica in that Arnica is more for the body of the muscles whereas Ruta is for the tendons and connective tissues. It has a particular affinity for the eyes and for joints, especially the wrist. Ruta is effective in relieving injury that results from overuse and is helpful in cases of eyestrain and repetitive strain injury.

SANGUINARIA
Sang
(Bloodroot)

Helpful for: Airborne allergens, Cluster, Food-related, Hypertension, Migraine, Mixed, Premenstrual, TMJ, Weather-related (sun)

Onset: Overexposure to sun. Overeating rich food or wine. Periodic (every third or seventh day).

Location: Primarily right-sided. Pain that begins in the back of head and spreads upward to settle over the eyes, especially the right eye or temple.

Sensation: Burning, bursting, as if eyes were being pressed out or head would explode. Lightning-like pain in the back of the head. Knifelike. Throbbing.

Modalities:
Better: Lying down. Sleep. Acidic foods and drinks. Firm pressure. Pain relieved by vomiting.
Worse: Right side. Motion. Touch. Daytime, pain rises and falls with the sun.

Concomitants: Face flushed, small red spots on cheeks. Eyes burn. Earache may accompany the headache. Palms of hands and soles of feet burn, as from hot water. Fullness and tenderness behind jaw hinges. Unquenchable thirst. Nausea with salivation and bilious vomiting.

Mentals & Generals: Angry and irritable, morose and grumbling. Gets sick and faint from the aroma of flowers. Loss of appetite. Craves spicy things, averse to butter and sugar. Sinking, "all-gone" feeling in stomach. Drowsy and indolent. Sleepless at night, can't sleep without brandy. Slight noises disturb sleep without fully arousing the sleeper.

Sanguinaria affects the vascular system, and its characteristic symptoms reflect disturbances in circulation. Burning sensations, a flushed face, and the throbbing pain associated with distended veins are typical. It is especially helpful for women who get headaches at specific times during their menstrual cycles or during menopause.

SPIGELIA
Spig
(Pinkroot)

Helpful for: Airborne allergens, Arthritis/cervical spondylitis, Cluster, Cold/Flu, Food-related, Migraine, Mixed, Rebound/caffeine, Tension, Trauma

CAUTION: Head injuries, or headache following an injury, *must* be evaluated by a medical doctor.

Onset: At sunrise. Taking cold.

Location: Left side. Front.

Sensation: Neuralgic pain: intense, shooting or pulsating, stitching, stabbing, or burning. Intolerable pain on moving the eyes. Eyes feel too large with the pain, intolerable.

Modalities:

Better: From noon to sunset. Lying with head propped up. Firm pressure on affected area. Rest. Dry air.

Worse: Daytime, especially from sunrise till noon. Motion. Stooping. Mental exertion. Eating. Noise. Cold, damp, rainy days. Light touch.

Concomitants: Hypersensitive to light and noise. Stiff neck and shoulders make moving painful. Pain in and around eyes and deep in the eye sockets. Eyes tear, especially on affected side. May have heart palpitations.

Mentals & Generals: Head pain worse with warmth and temporarily relieved by cold. Washing with cold water alleviates pain, but pain may be worse when you stop. (Other symptoms are better with cold, worse with heat.)

The patient is very restless and very anxious. If the pain is severe, he may be suicidal. He tries not to think about the pain; thinking about it makes him depressed. Typically the pain follows the course of a nerve. The patient can track the line of the pain; it is like a hot wire plunged into him. May feel like his skin is being torn off his face.

SULPHUR
Sulph
(Sublimated sulphur)

Helpful for: Airborne allergens, Cold/Flu, Exertion, Food-related (hunger or fasting), Migraine, Mixed, Rebound/analgesics, Rebound/caffeine, Trauma, Weather-related (sun)

CAUTION: Head injuries, or headache following an injury, *must* be evaluated by a medical doctor.

Onset: Sudden. From hunger or missed meals. Periodic, every 7 days.

Location: Left side. Top of head. Temples.

Sensation: Heat on the top of the head. Pounding, throbbing, beating headache. Burning. Heaviness, fullness, and pressure in head, especially the temples. Constriction.

Modalities:

Better: Warm room and applications, hot drinks, head uncovered.

Worse: At noon and midnight. Stooping, jarring, light, after eating, cold drinks, motion.

Concomitants: Flickering lights precede headache. Burning in palms of hands and soles of feet. Hands trembling, sweaty. Itching, worse with heat. Scratching causes burning. Skin is very sensitive, may avoid washing. Red, engorged face. Red eyes with tearing. Nose is dry and congested. Nausea and vomiting of bile. Knees and ankles stiff.

Mentals & Generals: Catnaps, rather than sleeping. Wakes at the slightest noise. Feels dull and stupid. Forgetful. Childish peevishness in adults. Selfish, no regard for others. Irritable, depressed, thin and weak (even with good appetite). Weak, faint, and hungry at 11 A.M. Inertia and feebleness of tone. Cannot walk erect, walks stoop-shouldered. Desires sweets or salt, but eating them aggravates the condition and may provoke nausea or vomiting.

Sulphur conditions are red, itching, and burning. They have a volcanic quality—they may lie dormant for long periods, then erupt suddenly and violently. Any discharges, including breath or sweat, may have an offensive odor. The kinds of ailments that respond to Sulphur exhibit symptoms of burning, redness, and sudden onsets—"eruptions" that may be literal, as in the sense of skin eruptions, or figurative in the suddenness of the appearance and disappearance of the symptoms. A common symptom is itching that is worse with warmth—especially the warmth of a bed at night—and aggravated by scratching (which may cause burning).

Remedy Charts

Remedy	Helpful for	Onset	Location	Sensation	Modalities >better <worse	Concomitants	Mentals & Generals
Aconite	Al, Cl, C/F, Ex, F-r, Hy, Mx, R/a, S, T, Tr	Sudden, violent. After a draft. Emotional shock.	Face & head.	Pain is "intolerable." Heavy. Hot, full. Pulsating. Bursting. As if skull were forced out of the forehead, or as if constricted by a tight band.	>Open air, still air. >Warmth, perspiring. <Evening, night. <Lying on affected side. <Tobacco smoke. <Light, noise.	Burning sensations. Fever. Dizziness. Thirst for cold drinks. Upset stomach. Diarrhea or constipation.	Great anxiety, fear, & worry out of proportion to the condition. Fear of imminent death. Restlessness.

Remedy	Helpful for	Onset	Location	Sensation	Modalities >better <worse	Concomitants	Mentals & Generals
Apis mellifica	Al, Ar, F-r, Hy, Mx, Pm, S, T, Tr	Emotional upset.	Back of head. Starts right, moves left.	Stinging, burning pain. Stabbing or piercing. Back of head, heavy, dull pain that extends to neck.	>Cold: applications, drinks/food, bathing. >Open air. >Pressure. <Heat: applications, drinks/food, bathing. <Lying down. <Motion. <In the afternoon, especially 3–5 P.M.	Head bent backwards or bored into pillow. Swelling, or the sensation of swelling. Skin flushed pink (not red). Stiffness. Thirstless, but may crave milk. Dizziness with sneezing.	Drowsy, listless, apathetic, indifferent. May start, scream, or cry out suddenly. May be whining, tearful, or irritable.

Al   Airborne allergens
Ar   Arthritis
Cl   Cluster
C/F Cold or flu

Ex   Exertion
Eye Eyestrain
F-r Food-related
Hg   Hangover

Hy   Hypertension
M   Migraine
Mx   Mixed
Pm   Premenstrual

R/a Rebound/Analgesics
R/c Rebound/Caffeine
S   Sinusitis
T   Tension

TMJ Temporomandibular Joint Syndrome
Tr   Trauma
W   Weather-related

Remedy	Helpful for	Onset	Location	Sensation	Modalities >better <worse	Concomitants	Mentals & Generals
Argentum nitricum	Cl, C/F, Ex, Eye, F-r, M, Mx, Pm, R/a	Gradual. Emotional upset. Mental exertion, especially with anxiety.	Left side. Front.	Head feels large; like bones are separating. Boring pain. Eye on affected side feels enlarged.	>Cold. >Fresh air. >Firm pressure, head wrapped with a tight band. <Heat. <At night. <During menstruation.	General debility. Coldness & trembling. Blurred vision, eyestrain, sensitive to light. Nausea, vomiting. Flatulence, belching.	Person feels better in fresh air, but headache may be aggravated. Melancholy. Nervous. Impulsive, feels time is passing slowly. Craves sweets, but eating them aggravates the condition.

Remedy	Helpful for	Onset	Location	Sensation	Modalities >better <worse	Concomitants	Mentals & Generals
Arnica	C/F, Ex, Eye, M, T	After injury (or an emotional "blow"). With a cold or the flu.	Generalized.	Bruised, sore as from a bruise. Head feels hot while body feels cold. Head feels contracted.	>Lying down. >Open air. >Warmth. <Least touch/ pressure. <Motion, exertion. <Damp, cold.	Dizziness, especially when walking. Eyestrain, with bruised feeling in eyes. Holds eyes open.	Wants to be left alone, fears being touched. Gloomy, irritable.
Arsenicum album	Ar, C/R, Ex, F-r, Hg, M, W	After exertion, excitement, or getting heated. 1–3 P.M. Periodic.	Forehead. Back of head. Right side.	Throbbing & burning. Waves of pain. Very chilly. Sick, severe headache. Congestion. Brain feels loose.	>Body warm & head cool. >Head elevated. >With company. <Heat. <Light, noise, motion. <At night (1–2 A.M.)	Exhaustion and restlessness. Nausea & vomiting, cannot bear the sight or smell of food. Pallor. Skin cold.	Anxious, restless. Seeks relief in motion. Fear, fright, worry. Sensitive to disorder & confusion.

Al	Airborne allergens	Ex	Exertion
Ar	Arthritis	Eye	Eyestrain
Cl	Cluster	F-r	Food-related
C/F	Cold or flu	Hg	Hangover

Hy	Hypertension	R/a	Rebound/Analgesics
M	Migraine	R/c	Rebound/Caffeine
Mx	Mixed	S	Sinusitis
Pm	Premenstrual	T	Tension

TMJ	Temporomandibular Joint Syndrome
Tr	Trauma
W	Weather-related

Remedy	Helpful for	Onset	Location	Sensation	Modalities >better <worse	Concomitants	Mentals & Generals
Belladonna	Al, Cl, C/F, Ex, Hy, M, Mx, S, W	Sudden, severe. Exposure of head to cold. Suppressing nasal mucus.	Right side. Front.	Throbbing, shooting, stabbing. Hot, burning. Heavy, full. Constricted, as though a band or strap were wrapped around the head. A rush of blood to the painful area.	>Warm wraps. >Bending head backwards. >Semierect posture. >Firm pressure applied gradually. <Light, noise, touch. <Cold & drafts. <Lying down. <Motion. <3 P.M. & 9 P.M.	Redness, flushed face. Dilated pupils. Dizziness when moving head. Blood in nasal mucous. Extremities ice-cold. Bores head into pillow, constant moaning.	Restlessness. Cries out or screams in sleep. Starts awake when falling asleep. Jerking & twitching. Senses hyperacute. Mental excitation. Furious, strikes out in a rage. Delirium, nightmares, may hallucinate. Disinclined to talk.

Remedy	Helpful for	Onset	Location	Sensation	Modalities >better <worse	Concomitants	Mentals & Generals
China officinalis	CI, C/F, F-r, M, R/a, Tr	Periodic, every other day	Back of head, base of skull.	As if skull would burst. Intense pain. Throbbing, may extend to the sides of the throat.	>Firm pressure. >Warm room. >Standing or walking. <Light touch, combing hair. Breezes. <After eating. <At night.	Visual disturbances. Ringing in the ears. Flushed face. Hunger with no appetite, full after a few bites. Slow digestion. Dizzy when walking.	Apathetic, indifferent, disobedient. Ill-tempered, hurts other's feelings. Insomnia, or unrefreshing sleep. Nightmares, with lingering fear of the dream. Sudden crying out. Restlessness.

Al	Airborne allergens	Ex	Exertion	Hy	Hypertension	R/a	Rebound/Analgesics	TMJ	Temporomandibular Joint Syndrome
Ar	Arthritis	Eye	Eyestrain	M	Migraine	R/c	Rebound/Caffeine	Tr	Trauma
Cl	Cluster	F-r	Food-related	Mx	Mixed	S	Sinusitis	W	Weather-related
C/F	Cold or flu	Hg	Hangover	Pm	Premenstrual	T	Tension		

Remedy	Helpful for	Onset	Location	Sensation	Modalities >better <worse	Concomitants	Mentals & Generals
Calcarea carbonica	Al, Ar, Ex, F-r, M, Mx, R/a, S, T, TMJ, W	Change of weather. Stress, mental exertion.	Right side. Radiating pain: forehead to nose, temples to jaw, muscles in back of neck to base of skull.	As if a heavy weight rested on top of the head. Scalp itches.	>Lying on painful side. >Dry climate and weather. <Any exertion. <Cold in any form. <Change in weather. <Wet weather. <Dampness in any form.	Eyes itchy, tearing. Night sweats. Cold hands and feet. Dizziness. Nausea. Large appetite with slow digestion. Craves eggs, averse to fats.	Insomnia, nightmares. Jaded, assumes too much responsibility. Apprehensive, may be afraid of the dark. Forgetful or slow-witted.

Remedy	Helpful for	Onset	Location	Sensation	Modalities >better <worse	Concomitants	Mentals & Generals
Bryonia	Ar, Cl, C/F, Ex, M, Mx, Pm, R/c, S, Tr	Slow, gradual. From cold. Upon awakening. Headache that precedes other complaints.	Base of skull. Front (& frontal sinuses) Right side.	Bursting. As if the skull would split open. Throbbing pain with slightest motion. Sharp stabbing pains over the eyes. Fullness & heaviness.	>Firm, steady pressure. >Lying down, may rest on painful side. >Lying still in a dark room. <Slightest motion, even moving the eyes. <Warm & stuffy room. <Sitting up. <Light. <After eating.	Feels sick & faint on rising or lifting head. Red congested eyes; soreness in eyeballs. Nosebleed. Runny nose with shooting and aching pains through forehead. Dryness. Thirsty. Constipation.	Must keep still. Peevish, wants to be left alone. Dull mind, slow, sluggish, passive. May feel homesick, even if at home.

Al	Airborne allergens	Ex	Exertion
Ar	Arthritis	Eye	Eyestrain
Cl	Cluster	F-r	Food-related
C/F	Cold or flu	Hg	Hangover

Hy	Hypertension	R/a	Rebound/Analgesics
M	Migraine	R/c	Rebound/Caffeine
Mx	Mixed	S	Sinusitis
Pm	Premenstrual	T	Tension

TMJ	Temporomandibular Joint Syndrome		
		Tr	Trauma
		W	Weather-related

Remedy	Helpful for	Onset	Location	Sensation	Modalities >better <worse	Concomitants	Mentals & Generals
Colocynthis	Al, C/F, F-r, Hy, M, Mx, Pm, S, T, W	After vexation. Hunger or fasting. Change of season.	Left side. Front.	Severe pain. Cramping, constriction, contraction. As if clamped with iron bands. Digging, rending, or tearing. Waves of pain.	>Firm pressure. >Resting with knees drawn up to chest. >Coffee. <Resting on back. <Stooping. <Moving eyelids. <Cold, damp weather.	Dizzy when turning head to the left. Nausea, vomiting. Bitter taste in mouth. Severe abdominal pain or cramping. Muscles cramped, joints stiff. Scalp sore. Burning tears.	Irritable, short-tempered. Angry. Indignant. Mortification from offense. May scream from the pain.

Remedy	Helpful for	Onset	Location	Sensation	Modalities >better <worse	Concomitants	Mentals & Generals
Ferrum phosphoricum	Ar, C/F, S, Tr, W	Sudden. Exposure to sun. From a cold or flu. From overexertion.	Right side. Forehead to base of skull, especially right side. Crown, sides.	Bruised, pressing, or stitching pain. Throbbing, pulsating. May feel a rush of blood to the head. Head hot & full.	>Cold air or applicatoins. >Lying down. >Pressure. <Night & early morning <Motion, jarring, stepping. <Light. Noise.	Stiff neck. Cheeks flushed. Nosebleed, bleeding gums. Feet cold. Dizziness. Cold symptoms: fever, runny nose, congestion, vomiting, body aches.	Sleep restless & dreamless. Night sweats. Talkative. Easily fatigued. Desires sour things. Thirst for cold water.

Al Airborne allergens
Ar Arthritis
Cl Cluster
C/F Cold or flu

Ex Exertion
Eye Eyestrain
F-r Food-related
Hg Hangover

Hy Hypertension
M   Migraine
Mx Mixed
Pm Premenstrual

R/a Rebound/Analgesics
R/c Rebound/Caffeine
S   Sinusitis
T   Tension

TMJ Temporomandibular Joint Syndrome
Tr   Trauma
W   Weather-related

Remedy	Helpful for	Onset	Location	Sensation	Modalities >better <worse	Concomitants	Mentals & Generals
Gelsemium	Ar, C/F, Eye, Hy, M, Mx, R/a, R/c, S, Tr, W	Gradual. Early morning. Emotional distress.	Back of head. Base of skull. Temples, extending to face.	Dull heavy ache. Great heaviness of eyelids and above eyes. A band of pain.	>Lying still, propped up with pillows. >Firm pressure. >After urination. >Fresh air. <Damp weather. <Emotional upset. <Mid-morning (10 A.M.). <Mental effort.	Profound exhaustion. Great weakness. Trembling. Nausea. Dizziness that spreads from the base of the skull. Eyes glazed, pupils dilated. Vision blurred. Neck & shoulders sore.	Drowsiness, dullness, apathy. Too exhausted to move or stand. Cannot stay awake. Groggy, lethargic.

Remedy	Helpful for	Onset	Location	Sensation	Modalities >better <worse	Concomitants	Mentals & Generals
Ignatia	Cl, C/F, F-r, M, Mx, R/a, R/c, S, T	Emotional distress: grief, disappoint- ment, anger.	Localized in one spot.	As if a nail has been driven into one spot. Head feels hollow & heavy.	>Firm pressure. >Bending forward. >After urination. <Strong odors, coffee, tobacco smoke. <Stooping. <Pressure on the painless side. <Morning.	Sensation of a lump in the throat. Vomiting. Chills with fever. Skin sensitive to draft.	Sad, brooding, tearful, rejects company. Light sleep or insomnia. Troubling dreams. Contradictory symptoms: nausea relieved by eating, eating increases hunger. Craves acid or indigestible foods.

Al Airborne allergens
Ar Arthritis
Cl Cluster
C/F Cold or flu

Ex Exertion
Eye Eyestrain
F-r Food-related
Hg Hangover

Hy Hypertension
M Migraine
Mx Mixed
Pm Premenstrual

R/a Rebound/Analgesics
R/c Rebound/Caffeine
S Sinusitis
T Tension

TMJ Temporomandibular Joint Syndrome
Tr Trauma
W Weather-related

Remedy	Helpful for	Onset	Location	Sensation	Modalities >better <worse	Concomitants	Mentals & Generals
Iris versicolor	Ex, F-r, M, Mx, R/a, R/c, T, Tr	After relief of stress. Periodic (every 4-6 weeks).	Front. Right temple.	Sick headaches. Scalp feels constricted. Nerve pains over entire face.	>Continued motion. >Cold drinks. <At night. <Rest.	Preceded by visual disturbances. Blindness during headache. Burning sensations. Acid vomiting.	Low-spirited, cranky, fault-finding. Unable to concentrate. Weak memory. Loss of appetite. Accelerated pulse. Chilly through the night.
Kalibichromicum	Al, Ar, C/F, M, Mx, R/a, S	Preceded by blurred vision.	Front. Sinuses in forehead and cheekbones.	Blinding headache. Migrating pain.	>Heat. Slightly>with pressure. <Morning. <Hot weather.	Thick, sticky, yellowish green mucus that is difficult to expel. Joint & low back pain. Coughing. Hoarseness. Stopped-up ears, earache.	Averse to light & noise. General weakness. No fever. Wakes up coughing or choking (from postnasal drip).

Remedy	Helpful for	Onset	Location	Sensation	Modalities >better <worse	Concomitants	Mentals & Generals
Lachesis	Cl, C/F, F-r, Hy, M, Mx, Pm, R/c, S, TMJ, Tr, W	Wakes from or with pain. From sun. In springtime.	Left side. Starts left, moves right.	Waves of pain. Throbbing, pulsating. Weight & pressure. Pressure & burning on the crown. Tearing pain in jaw.	>Onset of discharges, e.g., nasal mucus or menstrual flow. >Few clothes & no blankets. >Cool & cold temperatures. <Movement. <Light. Noise. <Light touch, pressure.	Senses are hyperacute. Congested head. Nosebleeds. Pale or mottled, purple face. Trembling. Dizziness, nausea & vomiting. Visual disturbances: weak vision, flickering, loss of sight.	Sleep aggravates condition. Very talkative. May not complete one thought before starting another. Melancholy, jealous, suspicious. Cannot stand the touch of clothes on the skin.

Al	Airborne allergens	Ex	Exertion	Hy	Hypertension	R/a	Rebound/Analgesics	TMJ	Temporomandibular Joint Syndrome
Ar	Arthritis	Eye	Eyestrain	M	Migraine	R/c	Rebound/Caffeine	Tr	Trauma
Cl	Cluster	F-r	Food-related	Mx	Mixed	S	Sinusitis	W	Weather-related
C/F	Cold or flu	Hg	Hangover	Pm	Premenstrual	T	Tension		

Remedy	Helpful for	Onset	Location	Sensation	Modalities >better <worse	Concomitants	Mentals & Generals
Lycopodium	Al, C/F, F-r, S, T	Gradual. Taking cold. Hunger or fasting. Congestion.	Right side. Starts right, moves left.	As if temples were screwed toward each other. Throbbing, pulsating. Pressure on crown. Tearing at base of skull.	>Motion. >Warm food or drink. >Cool air. <4–8 P.M. <Heat. Warm room or applications. <Noise. <Lying down.	Shakes head. Facial contortions. Gassy: belching and flatulence. Great hunger easily satisfied. Craves sweets, warm foods & drinks.	Nervous excitement & prostration. Wants to be alone, but wants to have someone nearby, if needed. Cranky on waking, may wake from hunger. Bullying. Fear of failure.

Remedy	Helpful for	Onset	Location	Sensation	Modalities >better <worse	Concomitants	Modalities >better <worse	Mentals & Generals
Magnesia phosphorica	Ar, C/F, F-r, M, Pm, R/a, S, Tr	Sudden, spasmodic.	Right side. Back of head. Over eyes, eyebrows.	Shooting, stinging, darting pain. As if brain were liquid, parts changing places. Eyes hot, vision blurred, colored lights before eyes.	>Always better with warmth. >Pressure, bending double. Rubbing.	Fever with chills. Shivering. Muscle cramps, radiating pain. Menstrual cramps.	<Right side. <Cold. <At night.	Languid, tired, exhausted. Constant lamenting about the pain. Sleepless due to indigestion.

Al	Airborne allergens	Ex	Exertion	Hy	Hypertension
Ar	Arthritis	Eye	Eyestrain	M	Migraine
Cl	Cluster	F-r	Food-related	Mx	Mixed
C/F	Cold or flu	Hg	Hangover	Pm	Premenstrual

R/a	Rebound/Analgesics	TMJ	Temporomandibular Joint Syndrome
R/c	Rebound/Caffeine	Tr	Trauma
S	Sinusitis	W	Weather-related
T	Tension		

Remedy	Helpful for	Onset	Location	Sensation	Modalities >better <worse	Concomitants	Mentals & Generals
Natrum muriaticum	Ar, Ex, Eye, M, M, R/a, R/c, S, T, Tr	Mid-morning (10 A.M.). Emotional distress: humiliation, grief. Eyestrain. Periodical.	Right eye. Back of head, extending down spine.	Blinding. Pounding, as if small hammers were knocking on the brain. Crushing, as if pressed in a vise.	>Open air. >Cold bathing. >Skipping meals. <Moving eyes. <Noise. <Heat, warm room. <Mental exertion, talking.	Mucous membranes dry. Lips parched, cracked. Tongue feels dry, like it sticks to the roof of the mouth. Nausea, vomiting. Visual disturbances. Stitching pains around eyes.	Craves salt. Must go to bed & be perfectly quiet. Depressed, discouraged, broken down. Tearful, but wants to be alone to cry. Cannot endure consolation. Insomnia.

Remedy	Helpful for	Onset	Location	Sensation	Modalities >better <worse	Concomitants	Mentals & Generals
Nux vomica	Ar/ Cl, C/F, Ex, F-r, Hg, M, Mx, R/a, R/c, Tr	After overindulgence in food, alcohol, or stimulants. Wakes with headache.	Back of head. Over eyes.	Splitting headache, as if a nail were driven into the crown. Sensation of a great weight on the crown. Frontal headache, with a desire to press head against something.	>Rest. >In the evening. >Wet weather. >Firm pressure. <In the morning. <Light, noise, smells. <Mental exertion. <Eating, overeating. <Stimulants, narcotics.	Pain with nausea & sour vomiting. Eyes dry, smarting, twitching. Sensitive to light. Back pain that is relieved by walking. Dizziness. Senses hyperacute.	Irritable, argumentative, and malicious. Sullen, faultfinding. Difficulty sleeping due to overactive mind or sensitivity to slight noises. Easily chilled; tends to avoid open air.

Al	Airborne allergens	Ex	Exertion	Hy	Hypertension	R/a	Rebound/Analgesics	TMJ	Temporomandibular
Ar	Arthritis	Eye	Eyestrain	M	Migraine	R/c	Rebound/Caffeine		Joint Syndrome
Cl	Cluster	F-r	Food-related	Mx	Mixed	S	Sinusitis	Tr	Trauma
C/F	Cold or flu	Hg	Hangover	Pm	Premenstrual	T	Tension	W	Weather-related

Remedy	Helpful for	Onset	Location	Sensation	Modalities >better <worse	Concomitants	Mentals & Generals
Pulsatilla	Al, F-r, M, Mx, Pm, R/a, R/c, S	Periodic. Premenstrual. After eating ice cream or rich foods. Overeating. Overindulgence. Overwork.	Right side. Forehead & sinuses.	Wandering, stitching pain through head & face, may extend into teeth. Pressure, distention, throbbing. Constricting, congestive.	>Cold: air, weather, food/drink, applications. >Slow motion in open air. >Pressure on painful side. >Onset of menses. <Evening and at night. <Lying or sitting still. <Motion of eyes. <Stooping.	Eyes itch. Profuse tears (especially on affected side) or bland yellowish discharge. Thirstless. Sour food causes vomiting.	Moody & changeable. Weepy, clinging. Averse to greasy food, warm food and drinks. Slow digestion, heartburn. Sleeps in the afternoon. May sleep with hands over head. Great desire for company, sympathy, consolation, reassurance of being loved.

Remedy	Helpful for	Onset	Location	Sensation	Modalities >better <worse	Concomitants	Mentals & Generals
Ruta graveolens	Al, Cl, Eye, Hg, R/c	After prolonged close work such as sewing or reading.	Eyes & eyebrows.	Pressure deep in eyes and over eyebrows. Eyes feel weary while reading. Stabbing, piercing as from a nail.	>Cessation of close work. >Heat. <Lying down. <Cold, wet weather.	Eyes are red, hot, tired. Blurry vision. Tearing. Nausea. Bones feel bruised. Neck or back pain.	Great restlessness. Lassitude, weakness. Tendency to despair. Self-dissatisfaction.

Al	Airborne allergens	Ex	Exertion	Hy	Hypertension	R/a	Rebound/Analgesics	TMJ	Temporomandibular Joint Syndrome
Ar	Arthritis	Eye	Eyestrain	M	Migraine	R/c	Rebound/Caffeine	Tr	Trauma
Cl	Cluster	F-r	Food-related	Mx	Mixed	S	Sinusitis	W	Weather-related
C/F	Cold or flu	Hg	Hangover	Pm	Premenstrual	T	Tension		

Remedy	Helpful for	Onset	Location	Sensation	Modalities >better <worse	Concomitants	Mentals & Generals
Sanguinaria	AI, Cl, F-r, Hy, M, Mx, TMJ, W	Sun. Overeating rich food or wine. Periodic (every third or seventh day).	Right-sided. Back of head to above right eye or temple.	Pain that migrates from base of skull & settles over the eyes. Bursting, as if head would explode. As if eyes were being pressed out. Knifelike, lightning-like pain in back of head.	>Lying down. >Sleep. >Firm pressure. >Acidic food/ drink. >After vomiting. <Daytime, rises & falls with the sun. <Motion. <Touch.	Palms & soles of feet hot, burning. Face flushed, small red spots on cheeks. Eyes burn. Fullness & tenderness behind jaw hinges. Nausea, salivation, & bilious vomiting.	Unquenchable thirst.

Remedy	Helpful for	Onset	Location	Sensation	Modalities >better <worse	Concomitants	Mentals & Generals
Spigelia	Al, Ar, Cl, C/F, F-r, M, Mx, R/c, T, Tr	At sunrise. Exposure to cold.	Left side, especially left eye, with tearing. Front.	Neuralgic pain: intense, shooting, pulsating, tearing, stitching, stabbing, or burning. Eyes feel too large, pain on moving eyes. Intolerable pain.	>From noon to sunset. >Lying with head high. >Firm pressure. <From sunrise till noon. <Mental exertion. <Eating. <Noise. Touch. <Cold, damp, rainy days.	Hypersensitive to light & noise. Stiff neck & shoulders. Pain in & around eyes & deep in sockets. Eyes tear, especially on painful side. May have heart palpitations.	Restless and anxious. If pain is severe, may feel suicidal. Pain follows a nerve. Washing with cold water relieves pain temporarily. (It returns when washing stops.)

Al	Airborne allergens	Ex	Exertion	Hy	Hypertension	R/a	Rebound/Analgesics	TMJ	Temporomandibular Joint Syndrome
Ar	Arthritis	Eye	Eyestrain	M	Migraine	R/c	Rebound/Caffeine		
Cl	Cluster	F-r	Food-related	Mx	Mixed	S	Sinusitis	Tr	Trauma
C/F	Cold or flu	Hg	Hangover	Pm	Premenstrual	T	Tension	W	Weather-related

Remedy	Helpful for	Onset	Location	Sensation	Modalities >better <worse	Concomitants	Mentals & Generals
Sulphur	A, C/F, Ex, F-r, M, Mx, R/a, R/c, Tr, W	Sudden. Hunger, missed meals. Periodic, every 7 days.	Left side. Top of head. Temples.	Heat on the top of the head. Pounding, throbbing, beating headache. Burning. Heaviness, fullness, pressure in temples. Constriction.	>Heat. Warm room & applications, hot drinks. >Head uncovered. <At noon & midnight. <Motion, stooping, jarring. <Light. <After eating. <Cold drinks.	Flickering lights precede headache. Burning in palms of hands & soles of feet. Itchy, worse with heat; scratching causes burning. Skin very sensitive, may avoid washing. Red face, red-rimmed eyes with tearing. Nausea & vomiting of bile.	Catnaps, rather than sleeping. Wakes at the slightest noise. Feels dull & stupid. Forgetful. Childish peevishness in adults. Irritable, depressed. Weak, faint & hungry at 11 A.M. Desires sweet or salt, but eating provokes nausea or vomiting.

Al	Airborne allergens	Ex	Exertion	Hy	Hypertension	R/a	Rebound/Analgesics	TMJ	Temporomandibular Joint Syndrome
Ar	Arthritis	Eye	Eyestrain	M	Migraine	R/c	Rebound/Caffeine	Tr	Trauma
Cl	Cluster	F-r	Food-related	Mx	Mixed	S	Sinusitis	W	Weather-related
C/F	Cold or flu	Hg	Hangover	Pm	Premenstrual	T	Tension		

PART FOUR

ADDITIONAL INFORMATION

Glossary

Acute Related to episodic stress or fatigue. Transient pain that can be related to particular precipitating factors, e.g., cold or flu, an injury, periodic stress.

Aggravation A temporary increase in the severity of symptoms due to taking a remedy in too high a potency.

Chronic A condition that is constant or recurs frequently (at least twice a week) and that resists treatment. Chronic conditions are often, but not always, genetically based. (*Note*: Chronic conditions should not be subject to self-care, but rather evaluated and treated by an experienced homeopath.)

Concomitants Secondary symptoms. Concomitant symptoms help identify appropriate remedies.

Dilution and succussion *See*: potentize.

Dose A unit of the remedy, usually 1–3 pellets or drops. (Also refers to the episode of taking the remedy.)

Generals A category of symptoms that includes eating and sleeping patterns, emotional states, and reactions to weather and interior environments.

Homeopathy A system for treating illness and injury with specially prepared substances, called remedies, that assist the body's efforts to heal itself. The remedies are taken singly, that is, one medicine at a time, in minute doses, and after careful assessment of a broad range of symptoms.

Homeopath Someone who practices homeopathy.

Law of cure A description of the progress of healing codified in the mid-1800s by Dr. Constantine Hering. His observations are that healing progresses from more vital organs and functions to less vital ones, that symptoms disappear in the reverse order from which they appeared, and resolve from top to bottom (that is head to feet).

Like cures like The primary tenet of homeopathy; in classic texts this idea is often given in Latin as: *similia similibus curentur.* It means that substances that can create symptoms in a healthy person can, when prepared according to homeopathic principles, aid the body in curing those symptoms in someone who is ill.

Location The site of the symptoms, illness, or pain.

Materia Medica Latin for "materials of medicine." A catalog of remedies detailing their effects.

Mentals Symptoms that affect the mental plane, for example: forgetfulness, poor concentration, confusion, or faulty perceptions of one's surroundings.

Minimal dosing The smallest effective dose of remedy. This idea is one of the four basic precepts of homeopathic philosophy.

Modalities A description of what makes you or your symptoms better or worse. These may include warmth or coolness, pressure on the painful area, sitting up or lying down, fresh air, motion or stillness, weather, and eating or drinking in general or eating and drinking particular things.

Onset A description of how the illness began, for example: rapid, gradual, after an injury, after exposure to weather.

Particular(s) The specific set of symptoms you develop

in reaction to an illness. Some of these are specific to the illness, for example, a cough or a stuffy nose with a cold; others are specific to the way you react to the illness. For example, you may wish to be left completely alone until you feel better and be irritable if disturbed, or you may have changes in your appetite or sleep patterns. The totality of your symptoms is matched against the remedy pictures to identify an appropriate remedy.

Peculiar(s) Symptoms that seem contradictory; for example, you may have chills but crave cold drinks, or you may have a frequent, urgent desire to urinate, but urinating is painful and scanty. In homeopathy, these unexpected combinations are often the most significant factors for determining an appropriate remedy.

Potentize Repeated dilution and succussion according to established homeopathic formulas to remove material components and isolate and activate the healing energy or vital force.

Provings An early form of clinical trials in which 100 healthy people were given a remedy and their reactions (symptoms elicited) were recorded. These records provided the source material for the Materia Medica.

Remedy A homeopathically prepared substance used to relieve illness. Remedies are available as pellets (a milk sugar base), as liquids, or as creams and gels.

Remedy picture The array of symptoms elicited in healthy people during a proving. These symptoms are cataloged in a materia medica and are the basis for recommending particular remedies for particular illnesses.

Repertory A reference book that details illnesses with their symptoms and suggests remedies that can alleviate them.

Repertorize The process of comparing a patient's symptoms against the illnesses cataloged in a repertory in order to recommend an effective remedy.

Succussion A portion of the process of preparing homeopathic remedies in which the substance is agitated by tapping, shaking, or stirring. Succussion alternates with dilution and is credited with maintaining the efficacy of the original substance despite extensive dilution.

Sensation The specific way the symptoms feel, for example, bursting, crushing, prickly, shooting, stabbing.

Symptoms The characteristic way that an illness manifests and the way in which you interact with the illness. Symptoms are the basis upon which remedies are recommended: The greater the consonance between the symptoms of the patient and the symptoms ascribed to the remedy, the more effective it will be.

Taking the case A diagnostic interview in which the homeopath asks a variety of questions to determine what your symptoms are in order to recommend an effective remedy. The interview may be short if the problem is an acute illness, such as a sore throat, or quite long (2–4 hours) if the illness is severe, complex, or chronic.

Totality of symptoms One of the basic precepts of homeopathy, and the one that best reflects its holistic base. Before recommending a remedy, a homeopath will ask for a "body scan"—a head-to-toe review of how you are feeling—and also ask about your mental, emotional, and spiritual reactions to the illness. This information, the totality of symptoms, determines the selection of remedies.

Vital force The energy that distinguishes animate from inanimate beings. Also, the active portion of a healing substance that is isolated by homeopathic dilution and succussion and instilled in the remedies.

Resources

Web site: Homeopathy Home Page
The homeopathy home page has searchable databases
of practitioners, professional organizations, pharmacies,
training programs, and veterinary institutions in the
United States and abroad.

http://www.homeopathy.com/directory/usa/
   organisations.html

Professional Associations, United States
These organizations maintain lists of qualified homeopaths and may provide referrals for a modest fee. Some
offer classes and other information suitable for laypeople.

American Association of Naturopathic Physicians
2366 Eastlake Avenue, Suite 322
Seattle, WA 98102
phone: 206 328 8510

National Center for Homeopathy
801 North Fairfax, Suite 306
Alexandria, VA 22314
phone: 703 548 7790
fax: 703 548 7792
website: www.homeopathic.org

North American Society of Homeopaths
122 East Pike Street, Suite 1122
Seattle, WA 98122
phone: 206 720 7000

Professional Associations, United Kingdom
British Homeopathic Association
   27A Devonshire Street
   London W1N 1RJ
   phone: 0171 935 2163

Council for Complementary & Alternative Medicine
179 Gloucester Place
London NW1 6DX
phone: 0171 724 9103
fax: 0171 724 5330

Society of Homeopaths
2 Artizan Road
Northampton NN1 4HU
phone: 01 604 621 400
fax: 01 604 622 622

Sources for remedies, United States
Some pharmacies and many health food stores carry
homeopathic remedies. The following companies distrib-
ute and/or manufacture homeopathic remedies. You may
buy individual remedies, combination remedies, or kits
that include several remedies for specific purposes, e.g.,

first aid, pediatric care. Some also sell instructional books and tapes.

Boericke and Tafel, Inc.
2381 Circadian Way
Santa Rosa, CA 95407
phone: 707 571 8202
fax: 707 571 8237

Boiron USA
6 Campus Blvd. Bldg. A
Newtown Square, PA 19073
phone: 800 BOIRON-1 (800 264 7661)
web site: http://www.boiron.fr

Dolisos America, Inc.
3014 Rigel Avenue
Las Vegas, NV 89102
phone: 800 DOLISOS (800 365 4767)

Homeopathy Works
124 Fairfax Street
Berkeley Springs, WV 25411
phone: 304 258 2541
fax: 304 258 6335
web site: www.homeopathyworks.com/index.htm

Luyties Pharacal Company
4200 Laclede Avenue
St. Louis, MO 63108
phone: 314 533 9600

Standard Homeopathic Company
P.O. Box 61067
204–210 West 131st Street
Los Angeles, CA 90061
phone: 800 624 9659

Resources for remedies, United Kingdom

Ainsworths
36 Cavendish Street
London W1M 7LH
phone: 0171 935 5330
fax: 0171 486 4313

Galen Homoeopathics
Lewell Mill,
West Stafford
Dorchester
Dorset DT2 8AN
phone: 01 305 263 996

Helios Homoeopathic Pharmacy
97 Camden Road
Tunbridge Wells
Kent TN1 2QR
phone: 01 892 536 393
fax: 01 892 546 850

Weleda (UK) Ltd.
Heanor Road,
Ilkeston,
Derbyshire DE7 8DR
phone: 01 602 309 319
fax: 01 602 440 349

Headache

For more information specific to headaches, contact the following agencies. Many hospitals have headache or pain clinics which can provide help and information for diagnosis and treatment.

American Association for the Study of Headache (AASH)
875 Kings Highway, Suite 200
West Deptford, NJ 08096
phone: 609 845 0322
fax: 609 384 5811

The Health Resource, Inc.
564 Locust Street
Conway AR 72032
phone: 501 329 5272
fax: 501 329 9489

National Headache Foundation
5252 North Western Avenue
Chicago, IL 60625
phone: 800 843 2256
(within Illinois: 800 523 8858)

Bibliography

Homeopathy

Pocket Manual of Homoeopathic Materia Medica
by William Boericke, MD
B. Jain Publishers Pvt. Ltd., 1990

Homeopathic Remedies for Health Professionals and Lay People
by Dale Buegel, Blair Lewis, and Dennis Chernin
Himalayan Publishers, 1978, 1991

Everybody's Guide to Homeopathic Remedies
by Stephen Cummings and Dana Ullman
Tarcher/St. Martin's Press, 1984

Organon of Medicine, 6th edition
by Samuel Hahnemann
translated by William Boericke, M.D.
B. Jain Publishers Pvt. Ltd. 1990

Repertory of the Homoeopathic Materia Medica
by J. T. Kent
B. Jain Publishers Pvt. Ltd., 1989

Homeopathic Medical Repertory: A Modern Alphabetical Repertory
by Robin Murphy
Hahnemann Academy of North America (HANA), 1993

Lotus Materia Medica: Homeopathic and Spagyric Medicines
by Robin Murphy
Lotus Star Academy, 1995

The Science of Homeopathy
by George Vithoulkas
Grove Press, 1980

Headache

Headache Free
by Roger Cady, M.D., and Kathleen Farmer, Psy. D.
Bantam Books, 1996

The Natural Health Guide to Headache Relief—The Definitive Handbook of Natural Remedies for Treating Every Kind of Headache Pain
by Paula Maas, D.O., M.D., (H.); Deborah Mitchell, and the editors of *Natural Health Magazine*
Pocket Books, 1997

Headache Relief
by Alan M. Rapoport, M.D., and Fred D. Sheftell, M.D.
Fireside/Simon and Schuster, 1990

Headache Help: A Complete Guide to Understanding Headaches and the Medicines that Relieve Them
by Lawrence Robbins, M.D. and Susan S. Lang
Houghton Mifflin, 1995

The Headache Book
by Seymour Solomon and Steven Fraccaro
Consumer Reports Books, 1991

HEALTH CARE BOOKS FROM KENSINGTON

EAT HEALTHY WITH KENSINGTON

COOKING WITHOUT RECIPES
by Cheryl Sindell   (1-57566-142-X, $13.00/$18.00)
Unleash your creativity and prepare meals your friends and family
will love with the help of this innovative kitchen companion. COOK-
ING WITHOUT RECIPES includes intriguing culinary strategies and
nutritional secrets that will stir your imagination and put the fun back
into cooking.

DINING IN THE RAW   (1-57566-192-6, $19.95/$24.95)
by Rita Romano
The first recipe book that explores high-enzyme living using raw
food cuisine. Complete with over 700 delicious recipes for entrees,
salads, soups, desserts, sauces and dressings, it explains how healthy
eating can actually help cure chronic ailments such as allergies, skin
disorders, arthritis, mood swings, colds, digestive problems and more
. . . *without* counting every calorie!

EAT HEALTHY FOR $50 A WEEK
Feed Your Family Nutritious, Delicious Meals for Less
by Rhonda Barfield   (1-57566-018-0, $12.00/$15.00)
Filled with dozens of recipes, helpful hints, and sample shopping
lists, EAT HEALTHY FOR $50 A WEEK is an indispensable hand-
book for balancing your budget and stretching your groceries while
feeding your family healthy and nutritious meals.

THE ARTHRITIC'S COOKBOOK
by Collin H. Dong, M.D.   (1-57566-158-6, $9.95/$12.95)
and Jane Banks
Afflicted with debilitating, "incurable" arthritis, Dr. Collin H. Dong
decided to fight back. Combining traditional Chinese folk wisdom
with his western medical practice, he created a diet that made his
painful symptoms disappear. Today, used in conjunction with regular
arthritis medications, this groundbreaking diet has provided thousands
of Dr. Dong's patients with active, happy, and virtually pain-free lives.
It can do the same for you.

*Available wherever paperbacks are sold, or order direct from the
Publisher. Send cover price plus 50¢ per copy for mailing and
handling to Kensington Publishing Corp., Consumer Orders,
or call (toll free) 888-345-BOOK, to place your order using
Mastercard or Visa. Residents of New York and Tennessee
must include sales tax. DO NOT SEND CASH.*

KEEP HEALTHY WITH KENSINGTON

ADVANTRA Z™   (1-57566-322-8, $5.99/$7.50)
The Natural Way to Lose Weight Safely
by Carl Germano, RD, CNS
Finally there's a natural way to stimulate weight loss, build lean muscle mass, and improve physical performance! This unique formula, derived from *Citrus Aurantium* (a Chinese herb used to stimulate healing), contains a rare composition of amines essential for turning your metabolism into a fat-burning mode. When used with a balanced diet and exercise, it also helps replace lumpy fat with sleek, powerful muscle. Whether you want to lose five pounds or fifty, or if you're a body builder and want that "cut" look faster, the mircale of Advantra Z™ has no potential side effects when used properly.

OLIVE LEAF EXTRACT   (1-57566-226-4, $5.99/$7.50)
by Dr. Morton Walker
This is Nature's antibiotic. A phenolic compound known as Oleuropein, extracted from the leaves of live trees is the source of powerful disease-resistant properties. Filled with case histories, testimonials and documented studies of diseases that were prevented, stabilized and some actually cured, this medical book will provide insight to information that can make you healthier. Strengthen your immune system, prevent viral diseases including HIV, herpes and the flu, eliminate symptoms of all types of infections, and even successfully treat the common cold . . . without side effects!

SHARK LIVER OIL   (1-57566-202-7, $5.99/$7.50)
by Neil Solomon, M.D., Ph.D., et al.
Sharks have an extraordinary resistance to infection. Studies have shown that shark liver oil has astounding healing and preventative effects on the human immune system. From helping you sleep better and fighting the common cold to lowering your blood pressure and raising your white blood and T cell count, this enlightening book will uncover the facts about this incredible immune strengthener.

Available wherever paperbacks are sold, or order direct from the Publisher. Send cover price plus 50¢ per copy for mailing and handling to Kensington Publishing Corp., Consumer Orders, or call (toll free) 888-345-BOOK, to place your order using Mastercard or Visa. Residents of New York and Tennessee must include sales tax. DO NOT SEND CASH.

PARENTING ADVICE

BABY: AN OWNER'S MANUAL
by Bud Zukow, M.D.   (1-57566-055-5, $14.00/$17.00)
If only babies came with their own instruction booklets. Well, Dr.
Bud Zukow has been fielding your most common (and not-so-
common) pediatric questions for more than 30 years. From
Ground Zero through the end of the First Year, this wise, witty,
indispensable book provides answers to your most pressing problems, and practical tips for getting you through the days and
nights.

HOW TO GET THE BEST PUBLIC EDUCATION
FOR YOUR CHILD   (0-8217-4038-5, $4.50/$5.50)
A Practical Parent's Guide For the 1990s
by Carol A. Ryan and Paula A. Sline, with Barbara Lagowski
The merits of public school are being questioned more fiercely
than ever before. Here is an insider's perspective combining general information with specific and practical advice, including how
to select the best school for your child, how to judge your child's
progress at school and how to evaluate your child's teacher. This
guide, by two authors with over 40 years of combined experience
in education, will help children fulfill their potential.

STEPPARENTING   (0-8217-4958-7,
$3.95/$4.95)
Everything You Need to Know to Make It Work
by Jeannette Lofas, CSW, with Dawn B. Sova
Practical, up-to-the-minute advice for dealing with the many baf-
fling issues that beset today's stepfamilies. From dating to remar-
riage, from stepsibling rivalry to joint custody, here is an invaluable
guide to coping with today's most complex challenge. Discover
the techniques, tools and strategies that break through the barriers.
Find creative solutions that can lead to happiness and success in
step relationships.

*Available wherever paperbacks are sold, or order direct from the
Publisher. Send cover price plus 50¢ per copy for mailing and
handling to Kensington Publishing Corp., Consumer Orders,
or call (toll free) 888-345-BOOK, to place your order using
Mastercard or Visa. Residents of New York and Tennessee
must include sales tax. DO NOT SEND CASH.*

THE MYSTERIES OF MARY ROBERTS RINEHART

THE AFTER HOUSE   (0-8217-4246-6, $3.99/$4.99)

THE CIRCULAR STAIRCASE   (0-8217-3528-4, $3.95/$4.95)

THE DOOR   (0-8217-3526-8, $3.95/$4.95)

THE FRIGHTENED WIFE   (0-8217-3494-6, $3.95/$4.95)

A LIGHT IN THE WINDOW   (0-8217-4021-0, $3.99/$4.99)

THE STATE VS.   (0-8217-2412-6, $3.50/$4.50)
ELINOR NORTON

THE SWIMMING POOL   (0-8217-3679-5, $3.95/$4.95)

THE WALL   (0-8217-4017-2, $3.99/$4.99)

THE WINDOW AT THE WHITE CAT
                          (0-8217-4246-9, $3.99/$4.99)

THREE COMPLETE NOVELS: THE BAT, THE HAUNTED
LADY, THE YELLOW ROOM
                        (0-8217-114-4, $13.00/$16.00)

Did you miss one?

Now you can buy these suspenseful books
From your favorite mystery authors...

GROSS JOKES
by Julius Alvin